Psychiatry Update 3

Series Editor
Michelle B. Riba, University of Michigan, Department of Psychiatry,
University of Michigan Eisenberg Family Depression Center
Ann Arbor, MI, USA

Psychiatry Update will encompass all areas of psychiatry research and clinical diagnosis and treatment. Chapters will publish randomly though out the year culminating in volumes throughout the year.

More information about this series at https://link.springer.com/bookseries/16222

Paula Riggs • Thida Thant
Editors

Cannabis in Psychiatric Practice

A Practical Guide

Springer

Editors
Paula Riggs
Department of Psychiatry
University of Colorado School of Medicine
Aurora, CO, USA

Thida Thant
Department of Psychiatry
University of Colorado School of Medicine
Aurora, CO, USA

ISSN 2524-8316 ISSN 2524-8324 (electronic)
Psychiatry Update
ISBN 978-3-031-04873-9 ISBN 978-3-031-04874-6 (eBook)
https://doi.org/10.1007/978-3-031-04874-6

This Springer imprint is published by the registered company Springer Nature Switzerland AG
The registered company address is: Gewerbestrasse 11, 6330 Cham, Switzerland

Foreword

Cannabis is not what it used to be.

Cannabis used to be underground. If you wanted to learn how terpenes affected your toke, how to hotbox a house party, or how to better the soil in your basement grow, you needed to know someone or purchase a specialist magazine. The knowledge you obtained was about an illegal substance whose cultivation, possession, and use were grounds for a felony. Today, cannabis is partially legal in many areas, where it is variously regulated as a medicine, an herbal product, a recreational substance, and, still, a Schedule 1 controlled substance. Today, knowledge can be obtained from a neighborhood cannabis dispensary which shares a shopping mall with grocery store where those cannabis specialist magazines are sold on the periodical aisle and cannabis derivatives are often available for sale a few aisles over among the beauty products, a late-capitalist definition of being aboveground.

Cannabis used to be a joint. If you wanted to use cannabis, most people smoked a low-potency, home-rolled cigarette. If you wanted something more, you needed a head shop to sell you a bong or vaporizer, or an experienced tinkerer who had figured out how to purify and compound cannabis into hash brownies and topical salves. Today, cannabis is available in a dizzying array of potencies from budtenders with varying degrees of credentials and experiences. Today, you can readily find recipes for cooking with cannabis and tutorials for turning cannabis into beverages, edibles, and oils instead of mere joints.

And yet, cannabis often remains the afterthought it has long been in medical education. Very few medical schools and training programs teach about cannabis or its use with the same rigor that they teach about alcohol, nicotine, and opiates, the other three of the four most commonly used psychoactive substances [1, 2].

In my medical training and psychiatric residency, I received few formal or informal teaching sessions about cannabis. In truth, I learned more about cannabis from my high school classmates than my med school faculty. I grew up in Colorado, a state where cannabis has long been the *de facto* state flower, with rates of cannabis use a figurative mile higher than the national average. I knew friends who began using in elementary school and as they did, I learned to associate their stoned behavior with the signature smell of the cannabis they smoked.

But it was only two decades later, after I began practicing as a physician, that I learned that the earthy, herbal smell I had long associated with cannabis was produced by the plant's dozens of terpenes, the aromatic oils which concentrate in the trichome crystals on a cannabis flower. I learned that knowledge from listening to my patients, meeting physicians engaged in Colorado's nascent medical cannabis system, and by reading the available literature.

There was little literature at the time. Searching PubMed, I found only thirteen studies of smoked cannabis, and no studies of edible preparations. Reading the studies as a physician, I was struck by the complexity of cannabis, with its dozens of psychoactive compounds, and the comparable simplicity of the literature. The published literature had small sample sizes, short durations, subjective outcomes, few active comparators, heterogenous populations, and modest outcomes. Worse, it excluded the high-potency formulations the people I met as patients were using [3]. That was in 2009, the year I completed residency, and the year aboveground dispensaries began appearing in Colorado. A year later, a third of all the cannabis dispensaries in the country were in Colorado, where two percent of the state's population had been registered to use cannabis for medical reasons, despite the still-limited evidence base [4].

My patients told me stories about benzoylindoles and BHO, salvia and Scooby Snacks, and tetrahydrocannabivarin and topicals. The language was as new to me, a mashup of biochemistry and slang, so I needed an interpreter.

I reached out to some of the physicians who were high-volume recommenders for the state's medical cannabis system. It was a small group. At that time, half of all the people registered to use medical cannabis in Colorado were enrolled by one of only twelve physicians. I asked one of them to teach me. He described the underground cannabis system and the medical cannabis system, often finding the former more social and the latter more professional. He would bring Twinkies infused with heroic amounts of Delta-9-tetrahydrocannabinol to our lunch meetings, but I am more of a nerd than a head, so I declined his samples and wrote research papers instead.

I found interested colleagues, so we wrote about a patient who attempted suicide after several episodes of heavy cannabis use [5], and then studied epidemiological associations between completed suicide and the cannabis registry [6]. We spent a year surveying hundreds of patients hospitalized in an adult psychiatric unit [7], and then studied the influence of cannabis use on psychiatric hospitalization outcomes [8].

None of those papers changed the world—research papers rarely do—but I learned a few things from them that I have tried to teach to other interested people [9, 10].

Cannabis means different things to different people. Some see it as a panacea, others as a poison. The first lesson was to move past slogans and seek evidence-based, but culturally humble, understandings of what cannabis means to people.

Cannabis means different things in different formulations. Some versions of cannabis appear to have effects equivalent to over-the-counter medications, while others can induce toxic syndromes. The second lesson was to give up generalities and be precise about the potency, dose, duration, formulation, and frequency of cannabis.

Cannabis means different things at different times. Some users will experience limited effects from cannabis, while others, especially children and adolescents, can experience enduring effects. The third lesson was that the use of cannabis is of greatest concern when use is started early in neurodevelopment and sustained over time, especially with high THC concentration formulations.

Cannabis means different things because it is differently regulated. For decades, it was impossible to conduct high-quality research studies because cannabis was a Schedule I substance, because they feared cannabis might be proven less harmful than their dire warnings. Today, one of the obstacles is the billion-dollar medical and recreational cannabis industries, which fear study because cannabis might be proven less beneficial than their advertisements. The fourth lesson was that cannabis should be regulated consistently across jurisdictions, without criminalization of use, and within a therapeutic relationship, so that we can truly understand what cannabis does for the people we meet as patients.

I take the work of the authors in this book, and their contributions, as a sign of cannabis' growth from the underground and into medical education. In these pages, you will find learned authors reflecting on their clinical experience and the available evidence. What you will not find is just as important: no scare tactics, no overpromising adverts. The authors offer an honest account of what cannabis is, what it does, and what it does not do. The book is necessary reading for any mental health clinician who wants to understand the substance that so many of our patients use. There are chapters on pharmacology, its effects on children and adolescents, presentations to consider in outpatient, emergency, and inpatient settings, and an account of how cannabis affects public health. Throughout, the authors provide clinical tips, high-yield tables, evidence-based references, and discuss the available psychotherapy and pharmaceutical treatments. In short, they offer evidence-based information in a single place, interpreted through the wisdom of clinical experience, that it would take a reader years to find only a decade ago.

Learning about the mental health effects of cannabis is not what it used to be. You can learn about it in a single book these days. For that change, I give thanks to the editors and authors of this collection.

Abraham M. Nussbaum

References

1. Evanoff AB, Quan T, Dufault C, Awad M, Bierut LJ. Physicians-in-training are not prepared to prescribe medical marijuana. Drug Alcohol Depend. 2017;180:151–5. https://doi.org/10.1016/j.drugalcdep.2017.08.010
2. Ware MA, Ziemianski D. Medical education on cannabis and cannabinoids: perspectives, challenges, and opportunities. Clin Pharmacol Ther. 2015;97(6):548–50. https://doi.org/10.1002/cpt.103
3. Borgelt LM, Franson KL, Nussbaum AM, Wang GS. The pharmacologic and clinical effects of medical cannabis. Pharmacotherapy. 2013;33(2):1950209.
4. Nussbaum AM. Ethical issues involving medical use of marijuana. Medical Ethics Advisor. 2013;29(9).
5. Nussbaum AM, Thurstone C, Binswanger IA. Medical marijuana use and suicide attempt in a patient with major depressive disorder. Am J Psychiatry. 2011;168(8):778–81.

6. Rylander M, Valdez C, Nussbaum AM. Does the legalization of medical marijuana increase completed suicide? Am J Drug Alcohol Abuse. 2014;40(4):269–73. https://doi.org/10.3109/00952990.2014.910520
7. Nussbaum AM, Thurstone C, McGarry L, Walker B, Sabel AL. Use and diversion of medical marijuana among adults admitted to inpatient psychiatry. Am J Drug Alcohol Abuse. 2015;41(2):166–72. https://doi.org/10.3109/00952990.2014.949727
8. Rylander M, Winston HR, Medlin H, Hull M, Nussbaum A. The association of cannabis use on inpatient psychiatric hospital outcomes. Am J Drug Alcohol Abuse. 2018;44(1):73–84. https://doi.org/10.1080/00952990.2017.1329313
9. Compton MT, American Psychiatric Association. Marijuana and mental health. 1st ed. Arlington, VA: American Psychiatric Association Publishing; 2016.
10. Thant T, Nussbaum A. What you need to know about cannabis: an evidence-based crash course for mental health trainees. MedEdPORTAL. 2020;16:10923. https://doi.org/10.15766/mep_2374-8265.10923

Series Editor Introduction

I live and work in Ann Arbor, Michigan, home to the University of Michigan and other great colleges and universities. For many years, it felt that as if there was a new coffee shop arising at just about every corner. That of course is an exaggeration. But recently, a new feeling pervades and is not an exaggeration—that there is a new marijuana shop on either a corner or ascending from a gas station!

Each state in the United States has its own history of cannabis legalization but in Michigan, medical use was legalized in 2008 through the Michigan Compassionate Care Initiative. In 2018, an initiative to legalize recreational use passed with a narrow margin. On December 1, 2019, licensed storefronts began adult-use retail sales.

It was always a routine question to ask patients about their use of alcohol, licit and illicit drugs, herbs, supplements, etc. with the prevalence of the use of marijuana in teens, college age students, and adults skyrocketing [1]. Marijuana is the most commonly used federally illegal drug in the United States with 48.2 million people or about 18% of the Americans having used it at least once in 2019 [1]. Further, studies are exploring the link or bidirectionality between marijuana and other gateway drugs like nicotine, alcohol, and cocaine [2].

Patients and families are increasingly asking questions about medicinal cannabis as well as recreational cannabis and its use related to psychiatric disorders. Patients are using cannabis for symptoms related to post-traumatic stress disorder (PTSD), anxiety disorder, depression, attention deficit hyperactivity disorder (ADHD), bipolar disorder, chronic pain, insomnia, opiate dependence, and schizophrenia as well as for neurological conditions such as the spasticity related to multiple sclerosis, agitation in dementia, and certain seizure disorders that are not well treated or managed by standard therapies. Further, cannabis is used to reduce symptoms such as nausea and anorexia related to cancer chemotherapies [3].

Understanding the pharmacology and biology of the various cannabis preparations, forms of use, interaction with psychotropic and other medications, and the exploding research are all critically important. Further we must be knowledgeable of the short-term and long-term risks and benefits of the use of cannabis, the various ways our patients are using the various preparations, and alert to various adverse effects and drug-drug interactions.

With all this in mind, we welcome this excellent text *Cannabis in Psychiatric Practice*.

This book is edited by Paula Riggs and Thida Thant, with thoughtful, knowledgeable authors who represent an interdisciplinary mix of colleagues who present us with up-to-date information that will serve to better equip us to partner with our patients and families in this burgeoning area of substance use. We welcome this book as the third volume in our Psychiatry Update Series and appreciate your review of this very important and useful text.

Most sincerely,
Michelle Riba, M.D., M.S.
Series Editor

References

1. Substance Abuse and Mental Health Services Administration. Key substance use and mental health indicators in the United States: Results from the 2019 National Survey on Drug Use and Health. Rockville, MD: Center for Behavioral Health Statistics and Quality, Substance Abuse and Mental Health Services Administration; 2020.
2. Lopez-Quintero, et al. Probability and predictors of transition from first use to dependence on nicotine, alcohol, cannabis, and cocaine: results of the National Epidemiologic Survey on Alcohol and Related Conditions (NESARC). Drug Alcohol Depend. 2011;115(1–2):120–30.
3. Fichtner CG, Moss HB. Medical marijuana and mental health: cannabis use in psychiatric practice. Psychiatric Times. 2017;34(5):1–8.

Preface

Lately, it occurs to me What a long, strange trip it's been
—Grateful Dead, *Truckin'*

These lyrics were the first to come to mind when asked about my experience, as a Child & Adolescent, Adult, and Addiction Psychiatrist, with the ever-expanding commercial environment of legalized marijuana over the past decade. As a Professor and Director of the Division of Addiction Science, Prevention and Treatment in the Department of Psychiatry at the University of Colorado School of Medicine, I felt it was my responsibility to be informed and to inform others about current research on the impact of cannabis use on health and mental health. Over the past decade I have been asked to speak on this topic at numerous public health forums, local and national radio and television interviews, and national scientific meetings. I also served on state policy and advisory boards to determine the safety labeling of commercial cannabis products and to review applications for state-funded cannabis research projects. Taken together, what have I learned from these experiences?

First, the political and economic drivers of the cannabis industry are often misaligned with efforts to promote dissemination of accurate scientific information. There remains much misinformation about cannabis in the public domain, making it difficult for many to distinguish research-based information from unsubstantiated claims. Second, given the rapid and ongoing national expansion of the legalized cannabis environment, there is an urgent need for more rigorous research on the health effects of cannabis use across the lifespan. Third, it is imperative for physicians and other healthcare clinicians to stay abreast of this research to inform their clinical practice and accurately inform patients and families. It is our hope that this volume will significantly contribute to this effort.

Aurora, CO — Paula Riggs

Introduction and Acknowledgements

I think it is an understatement to say that cannabis use is a controversial topic across the United States. Opinions about cannabis range from it being a harmless natural plant with medicinal value to a substance of abuse. Despite the classification of cannabis on a federal level, cannabis use is becoming legalized by states across the United States.

Transitioning from Texas to Colorado during medical training was a culture shock as far as cannabis is concerned. To the extent that cannabis was taught in medical school (i.e., it is automatically a use disorder since it is illegal), I was left woefully underprepared for what I would face in psychiatry training. Patients came into the office requesting medical cards; they could run circles around me when discussing strains and "indications" for use.

As my time in Colorado went on, I began to develop an expertise in the impact of marijuana use on psychiatric practice, disorders, treatments, et cetera, in a state with both recreational and medical marijuana. As I met more and more clinicians facing increasing cannabis use in their practices, I saw they had the same questions, lack of training and comfort that I initially had. It has become clear that with the increasing prevalence and availability of cannabis and CBD products, psychiatrists will need to become more well versed about cannabis beyond the scope of addiction and be able to discuss the existing literature and knowledge effectively with patients.

Many cannabis books to date are organized largely by disorder or symptom. *Cannabis in Psychiatric Practice: A Practical Guide* will be organized by clinical setting to help tailor the literature to psychiatrists working in all areas, whether traditional outpatient clinics, emergency departments, inpatient psychiatry, or medical units. This will help readers, regardless of their training background, learn about the impact of cannabis on a variety of disorders in a manner adjusted to the unique needs and challenges of their particular treatment settings and patient populations.

Some topics of particular importance will receive a dedicated chapter (such as psychosis) though others will be addressed in multiple chapters based on setting. Some chapters will include more basic science for the scientists at heart (the pharmacology chapter and neurodevelopmental chapter in particular) with most chapters designed for the busy general clinician. Clinical cases and practical tips integrating the current state of evidence, treatment approaches, and psychoeducation will be included.

Another important caveat is that while both authors and editors strive to make our recommendations as evidence and research based as possible, the current legal status of cannabis (and subsequently the quality of associated research) makes this extremely difficult. When possible, we present an overview and rating of the evidence. In more gray areas, we present an approach to clinical care, including assessment of the patient, considerations for treatment, evaluation of the existing evidence, and how to weigh the risks and benefits based on the expertise of our authors and their extensive experience practicing in states with "legalized" cannabis.

We start this book off with a bird's eye view of cannabis including an overview of legalization and public health concerns such as the medical, legal, and economic impact by Dr. Anna McDowell. In Chap. 2 Dr. Andrew Kluemper provides an overview of cannabinoid-related pharmacology (pharmacokinetics, drug-drug interactions, formulations, side effects) and the endocannabinoid system followed by a more in-depth dive into CBD by Dr. Susan Weiss and Dr. Katia Howlett in Chap. 3. The child and adolescent portion of the book begins with a more technical overview of the neurodevelopmental impacts of cannabis on the developing brain by Dr. Jesse Hinckley and Dr. John Dillon in Chap. 4 and then in Chap. 5 transitions into how to approach evaluation and treatment of cannabis use in the outpatient child and adolescent mental health setting by Dr. Paula Riggs. Chapter 6 by Dr. Gautam Rajendran and I reviews the evaluation and treatment of cannabis use and its effect in the acute psychiatric setting (emergency room and inpatient) while in Chap. 7 Dr. Beau Carubia and Dr. Anne Penner review consultation-liaison specific psychiatric concerns in acute pediatric medical settings. We then shift into the adult psychiatry portion of the book, starting with Dr. Matthew Shirazi and Dr. David Riedford reviewing the impact of cannabis use on the disease course and prognosis of a variety of disorders including mood disorders, anxiety disorders, PTSD, and ADHD in Chap. 8. In Chaps. 9 and 10, Dr. Alexis Ritvo and Dr. Sirish Veligati guide us through evaluation and management of concurrent cannabis use and mental health disorders in the adult outpatient setting. In Chap. 11, Dr. Scott Simpson and Dr. Peter Gooch take us into the psychiatric effects of cannabis in the acute psychiatric setting (emergency department and inpatient) with a focus on agitation and violence. Chapter 12, written by Dr. Ryan Lawrence and Dr. Ina Becker, focuses on cannabis and psychosis. Dr. Thom Dunn provides Chap. 13 on the impact of cannabis use on self-harm and suicide. In Chap. 14, Dr. Heather Murray and I present on effects of cannabis in the adult consultation-liaison/medical setting including delirium, medical catatonia, withdrawal, and cannabis hyperemesis. We then shift to the final section of the book and "special" populations. Chapter 15, provided by Dr. Sarah Nagle-Yang and Dr. Parvaneh Nouri, reviews particular considerations of cannabis use in the peripartum period including impact on lactation, legal concerns, screening methods, and epidemiology. Chapter 16, by Dr. Helena Winston, focuses on effects in the geriatric population including on cognition, driving, falls, and most common reasons for use (such as insomnia and pain). Chapter 17, our final chapter by Dr. Scott Winder and Dr. Erin Clifton, focuses on issues in the solid organ transplant population, including logistical, legal, and ethical matters and evaluation approaches.

Our hope is that this book will suit all learning styles, from those who like to read a book from cover to cover, to those who prefer to "spot" read pertinent sections. Information will be presented for both clinician and patient alike with the goal of improving collaborative, well-informed, and evidence-based decision making. Understanding cannabis across the lifespan is also incredibly important, and we made sure to cover the full range in this book, from perinatal exposure to geriatrics. We also included a few "special populations" chapters for those working in more specialized settings. In short, in our book we hope that you are able to find at least an introduction to any clinically salient area of cannabis in psychiatry.

I am deeply indebted to all the busy clinicians that contributed to this book. Taking the time to write a chapter on top of busy clinical schedules is never easy and this task was further complicated not only by the breadth (or frequently lack) of research and literature to review but also by the emotional, physical, and other tolls of the COVID-19 pandemic. To be concise, unbiased and high yield is more challenging than not, and I am appreciative of the time, effort, and flexibility of all involved.

Thida Thant

Contents

Contributors

Ina Becker Department of Psychiatry, Columbia University Medical Center, New York, NY, USA

Comprehensive Psychiatric Emergency Program, New York-Presbyterian Hospital, New York, NY, USA

Beau Carubia Department of Psychiatry, Children's Hospital Colorado, University of Colorado School of Medicine, Aurora, CO, USA

Erin G. Clifton Department of Psychiatry, University of Michigan, Ann Arbor, MI, USA

John Dillon Department of Psychiatry, University of Colorado School of Medicine, Aurora, CO, USA

Thom Dunn Behavioral Health Services, Denver Health, Denver, CO, USA

Psychological Sciences, University of Northern Colorado, Greeley, CO, USA

Peter Gooch Goucher College, Baltimore, MD, USA

Jesse D. Hinckley Department of Psychiatry, University of Colorado School of Medicine, Aurora, CO, USA

Katia Delrahim Howlett Division of Extramural Research, National Institutes of Health, National Institute on Drug Abuse, Bethesda, MD, USA

Andrew Kluemper Pharmacy Department, University of Colorado Hospital, Aurora, CO, USA

Ryan E. Lawrence Department of Psychiatry, Columbia University Medical Center, New York, NY, USA

Comprehensive Psychiatric Emergency Program, New York-Presbyterian Hospital, New York, NY, USA

Anna McDowell Mental Health Service, Rocky Mountain Regional Veterans Affairs Medical Center, Aurora, CO, USA

Heather Murray Department of Psychiatry, University of Colorado School of Medicine, Aurora, CO, USA

Sarah Nagle-Yang Department of Psychiatry, University of Colorado Anschutz, Denver, CO, USA

Parvaneh Nouri Department of Psychiatry, University of Colorado Anschutz, Denver, CO, USA

Anne Penner Department of Psychiatry, Children's Hospital Colorado, University of Colorado School of Medicine, Aurora, CO, USA

Gautam Rajendran Children's Hospital Colorado, Aurora, CO, USA

David Riedford Department of Psychiatry, University of Colorado School of Medicine, Aurora, CO, USA

Paula Riggs Department of Psychiatry, University of Colorado School of Medicine, Aurora, CO, USA

Alexis Ritvo Department of Psychiatry, University of Colorado School of Medicine, Aurora, CO, USA

Matthew Shirazi Department of Psychiatry, UCHealth Medical Center of the Rockies, University of Colorado School of Medicine, Fort Collins, CO, USA

Scott A. Simpson Behavioral Health Services, Denver Health and Hospital Authority, Denver, CO, USA

Thida Thant Department of Psychiatry, University of Colorado School of Medicine, Aurora, CO, USA

Sirish Veligati Department of Psychiatry, University of Colorado School of Medicine, Aurora, CO, USA

Susan R.B. Weiss Division of Extramural Research, National Institutes of Health, National Institute on Drug Abuse, Bethesda, MD, USA

Gerald Scott Winder Department of Psychiatry, University of Michigan, Ann Arbor, MI, USA

Department of Surgery, University of Michigan, Ann Arbor, MI, USA

Helena Winston Department of Psychiatry, University of Colorado, School of Medicine, Aurora, CO, USA

Denver Health, Denver, CO, USA

Public Health Concerns of Cannabis

1

Anna McDowell

Introduction

Many people in the U.S. use cannabis. In this chapter we will review the epidemiology of use, a brief history of cannabis legalization, and a review of the current status of legalization. The public health impact of cannabis use will be discussed as well as the legal and economic impact of cannabis use to date, as an increasing number of states move towards increased legalization and permissibility of use.

Epidemiology and Review of Legalization in the U.S.

Cannabis is the second most commonly abused psychoactive substance in the U.S., after alcohol, with approximately 13% of the population using cannabis in 2016 [1]. More men than women report using cannabis [2]. Potency is increasing, with consequential increases in degree of intoxication and users who are likely to develop use disorder [3]. Accidental exposures in children are increasing [4]; intentional, and illegal, use in adolescents has largely remained stable [5]. Pregnant and nursing women are more likely than ever to use cannabis [6], as are older adults [7]. Such increased use correlates with increasing legalization to varying degrees in the U.S. All states except Idaho, Nebraska, and Kansas have legalized recreational, medical, and/or cannabidiol (CBD)-low delta-9 tetrahydrocannabinol (THC) concentration cannabis use as of 2021. See Fig. 1.1 for a detailed map of State Cannabis Programs as of March 2021.

Reflecting the ever-changing legalization by states of cannabis use, in November 2020, voters in Mississippi and South Dakota voted to approve regulated medical use;

A. McDowell (✉)
Mental Health Service, Rocky Mountain Regional Veterans Affairs Medical Center, Aurora, CO, USA
e-mail: anna.mcdowell@va.gov

P. Riggs, T. Thant (eds.), *Cannabis in Psychiatric Practice*, Psychiatry Update 3,
https://doi.org/10.1007/978-3-031-04874-6_1

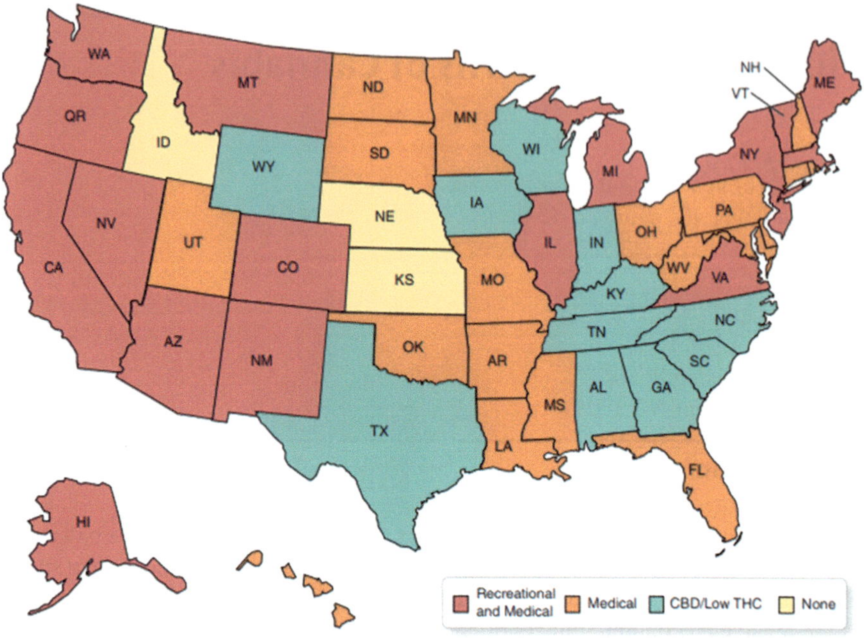

Fig. 1.1 State Cannabis Programs as of March 2021

there is a pending court challenge to the Mississippi measure. Similarly, voters in Arizona, Montana, and New Jersey approved recreational use while both New Mexico and Virginia lawmakers have passed bills legalizing recreational use which await their respective governors' (anticipated approving) actions. Conversely, though South Dakota voters approved an amendment to legalize adult recreational use in November 2020, on February 7, 2021, the Circuit Court deemed the amendment unconstitutional resulting in adult recreational use remaining illegal in South Dakota [8].

Medical cannabis use has been legalized in at least some states since California first legalized medical use in 1996 [9]. Of note, medical cannabis legalization routinely predates adult recreational use legalization. All but 14 states have a medical cannabis program. State medical programs vary significantly in how patients are recommended, or "prescribed," cannabis, how patients then obtain cannabis (e.g., growing of plants at home v. buying products at a dispensary), and how or even if patients are followed by the originally evaluating medical provider. The indications for medical cannabis program enrollment also vary by state with most states listing at least severe pain, spasticity, nausea, and cachexia as qualifying indications, though the variety of qualifying indications varies significantly from state to state. Further, some states list mental health diagnoses, such as Posttraumatic Stress Disorder, as indications for medical cannabis use despite lack of robust evidence [10]. The most common chief complaint of the patient seeking enrollment in a medical cannabis program has been found to be "chronic or severe pain," which is usually noted by patient self-report only [11, 12]. In fact, there remains a question as to the degree of overlap in characteristics of medical users of cannabis and recreational users of cannabis.

The first states to legalize recreational cannabis were Colorado and Washington, both, via citizen vote in November 2012; medical use of cannabis was legalized in each state in 2000 and 1998, respectively. As of the writing of this chapter, 15 states and the District of Columbia have legalized adult recreational use of cannabis (noting that some localities are still in the implementation phases of legalization). Legalization differs from decriminalization, or the reduction of statutory penalties for use-related acts, including personal possession, which started in Oregon in 1973 [13] and is now established in 27 states at the District of Columbia [8]. The degree of decriminalization varies by location, with Washington state as an example where possession of small amounts of cannabis and private use have been legalized for some time though citizens can still be legally penalized for growing plants at home. It must be noted that the enforcement of laws regarding cannabis, as well as other substance use, unfortunately may vary significantly by local police and legal jurisdiction.

Medical Impact: Special Populations

Exposure of children to cannabis is largely described as, and found to be, unintentional. In states following legalization, Emergency Department presentations significantly increased despite some states requiring explicit warnings on packaging [14]. Sudden onset lethargy and ataxia are common presenting complaints, as well as tachycardia, mydriasis, and hypotonia. Though hospitalizations of children after cannabis ingestion are typically brief and deaths have not been reported, a small number of children have required intubation [15]. The National Poison Data System reports increasing calls for CBD-containing products with notable increases reported from 2018 to 2020, 43% of all calls for children <5 years old, and 92% of all cases occurred in a residence [16]. Taken altogether, this highlights the need for continued education and awareness of the dangers of accidental ingestion of cannabis-containing products in children.

Unlike in children, adolescent exposure is usually intentional, more likely to be repetitive, and always illegal. As noted above, adolescent exposure to cannabis has largely remained stable or decreased, correlating with tobacco use and tobacco cessation public health efforts. Adolescent cannabis use has been found to correlate with poor educational outcomes, cognitive impairment and lower IQ, lower life satisfaction and achievement, and addiction [9]. However, without assessment of pre-cannabis use function and in the likely presence of confounding risk factors, these findings have not been determined to be conclusive. Regarding mental health diagnoses, adolescent cannabis use has been found to correlate with the development of schizophrenia spectrum disorders [17] and potentially exacerbate symptoms of mania [18]. Further research is needed to assess any causality; however, it is relatively safe to conclude that cannabis use in the developing brain is unlikely to be helpful. This point is discussed in more depth in Chap. 4, "Developmental Impact."

Use of cannabis by the pregnant or nursing woman has also been shown to have negative effect on the developing fetal brain and growing infant brain, respectively. Though briefly reviewed here, please see Chaps. 4, "Developmental Impact," and 15, "Cannabis in the Perinatal Period," for more details. Pre- and postnatal exposure has been found to correlate with low birth weight, reduction in head circumference, cognitive deficits (attention, learning, memory), disturbances in emotional response (leading to aggressiveness, high impulsivity, or affective disorders), and higher risk to develop substance use disorder [19]. Though there is opportunity for prenatal intervention at the many prenatal appointments women are recommended to attend, postnatal intervention opportunities are somewhat more limited as inquiry into infant feeding beyond "formula or breastmilk?" is rare. With THC evident in breastmilk as soon as 1 h after use and detectable as many as 6 days after last use [20], this is an area ripe for intervention.

Older adults make up another specific cohort of the population that is demonstrating increased cannabis use [7]; please see Chap. 16, "Cannabis in the Geriatric Population," for more information. There are many potential reasons for this, one being that cannabis use is known to be higher in patients with medical problems [21]. This is concerning for a number of reasons including older patients are more susceptible to side effects from cannabis use including confusion, dizziness and falls, and delirium.

Interestingly, cannabis use in the general adult population has not to date been reported to be related to an increased risk of death [22] though cannabis has been implicated indirectly in overdose and suicide deaths [23, 24], and at least one study has suggested cannabis is implicated in cases of cardiovascular and cerebrovascular death after use [25]. Despite the absence of evidence that cannabis is a cause of death, cannabis use is known to increase the risk of motor vehicle accidents, both fatal and nonfatal [26, 27], with cannabis users also being less likely to wear seatbelts [28]. Blood levels of THC 2–5 ng/ML have been indicated as causing impairment and especially in those who do not smoke regularly [29]. It should be noted, however, that THC levels for cannabis use are not equivalent to blood alcohol concentration for alcohol use as presence of cannabis metabolites in blood, urine, or saliva does not always correlate with recent use or intoxication. Many states are developing roadside assessment tools as well as behavioral assessment tools for apprehending the driver under the influence of cannabis.

Medical Impact: Emergency and Hospital Patients

Presentation of adults to the emergency department secondary to cannabis use has increased with the increase in states with legalization and medical use [30]. Visits to the medical ED for cannabis hyperemesis syndrome, gastrointestinal complaints [31], intoxication, and psychiatric complaints are common [32]. Regarding mental health specifically, cannabis use is known to exacerbate anxiety, psychotic symptoms and even psychotic disorders, as well as suicidal ideation [33]. Cannabis use is often noted in patients who struggle with other substances of abuse; Cannabis Use Disorder is rarely reported as a sole mental health diagnosis [34]. Similarly and contrary to popular belief, cannabis users can indeed develop physiological dependence on cannabis [35]. Though investigators continue to explore cannabis as a treatment option for a number of mental illnesses, outcomes thus far have not been promising [36].

In hospitalized patients, cannabis abuse is increasing, especially among older patients as well as medically ill patients with disability. Despite this, the most common primary conditions associated with cannabis use were psychiatric disorders and alcoholism [37]. Another study looked at opioid pain reliever-related hospitalizations in states with medical marijuana policies [38]. They found that states with medical marijuana policies had fewer opioid pain reliever-associated hospitalizations though no difference in marijuana-associated hospitalizations. Both studies suggest that cannabis use, though pursued as a medical panacea, is rarely without its own consequences.

In specific hospital populations, there is an increasing percentage of burn patients who have positive cannabinoid levels on hospital admission [39]. Similarly, increasing number of transplant candidates are using cannabis. Transplant outcomes thus far have not found differences in survival rates among kidney, liver, lung, and heart transplant recipients, though an increase in transplant complications with cannabis use has been noted [40]; Chap. 17, "Marijuana Use in Organ Transplantation," has a helpful discussion of this topic. Our understanding of the complicated interplay of cannabis use and medical recovery continues to evolve; it is recommended that clinicians caring for the medically ill patient, as with all patients, take into account the complex influence of social factors in collaborating with patients on treatment goals.

Legal Impact

Cannabis remains illegal under federal law yet remains the most commonly used illicit substance. A direct cause of this is the ready availability of cannabis in all 50 states, regardless of the degree of legalization. Cannabis is commonly diverted from legal markets in a variety of ways, including medical growers selling what they do not use, state-licensed growers selling portions of their product on the black market for higher rates, and some growers shielding illegal grow operations behind the Hemp Farming Act of 2018 which allows for farming of hemp as long as delta-9 tetrahydrocannabinol concentration is not more than 0.3% of the dry weight of the plant [41].

The potential profit from selling the harvest from even a small number of marijuana plants should not be dismissed. An experienced grower can produce up to 1 pound of cannabis in a 90-day growing cycle. The black market rate for high-quality cannabis is $800–$1000/pound, equaling $12,000 per year from just one plant; most growers selling to the black market will have yields from more than one plant [41].

Aside from the hypothetical small grower, medical licensee, and state-licensed growers selling illicitly for profit, it must be remembered that cannabis is an illegal drug that is traded with other illegal drugs by drug trafficking organizations and transnational criminal organizations. Cannabis is used in money laundering and often trafficked with other illegal substances. Seizures have been reported with illegal opioids, methamphetamine, guns, as well as large amounts of cash [41].

While it is challenging to find aggregate national data on the legal impact of cannabis decriminalization and legalization, the state of Colorado, being one of two states who legalized recreational cannabis use first in 2012 along with Washington State, can provide a snapshot of the legal impact of recreational cannabis use. The Rocky Mountain High Intensity Drug Trafficking Area compiled an aggregate report on the impact of cannabis legalization in Colorado [42]. Interestingly, and as noted above, there continues to be a high rate of Black Market seizures in Colorado. Most of these are illegal large-scale grow situations developed with the goal of selling product at higher prices in states where cannabis is still illegal.

Relating to impact on crime in Colorado, one study found that the presence of even one dispensary in a neighborhood increased neighborhood crime and disorder, including robbery and aggravated assault. The rate of murder in Denver did not increase over the time period studied; the rate of drug-related offenses did [43]. Another study looked specifically at crime near recreational versus medical dispensaries in Colorado. The authors found the property and drug crimes near recreational dispensaries increased, while property and drug crimes near medical dispensaries did not increase and even decreased in some areas, though not to a level of significance. No difference in the rate of violent crimes was observed [44]. The authors went further to also calculate the cost ratio of the increase in crime to the tax revenue, discussed further below, and found that for every $1 cost in crime, the tax revenue was $1.18. It remains to be seen if continued legalization efforts will yield a net gain in the communities that are dealing with the negative consequences of legalization.

Economic Impact

Marijuana continues to be the most commonly detected illegal substance in all workforce settings and specimen types with positivity frequency increasing 29% from 2015 to 2019 [45]. While difficult to find specific numbers in the workforce, highly publicized firings in 2021 of 5 White House Staffers relating to past cannabis use highlight the continued divide between both state and federal permissibility of cannabis use as well as the unclear expectations for employees who live in states with legalized and/or medical cannabis laws.

The majority of states that have legalized recreational or medical cannabis use leave drug testing and expectations regarding use to the employer. Twelve states and the District of Columbia have passed antidiscrimination measures for medical cannabis uses. Nevada is the only state that also passed accommodation for medical cannabis users as well as recreational cannabis-use antidiscrimination measures [8]. It should be noted that even in states where medical or recreational cannabis is legalized, the state supreme courts, when tested, have consistently determined that federal law supersedes state law.

Regarding revenue, U.S. states reported a combined $7.1 billion in tax revenue from marijuana sales as of February 2021, excluding locality-imposed taxes as allowed in some states. Tax rates vary by state, generally from 10% (many states tax 10–15%) to 37% (in Washington), excluding sales tax [46]. Some states additionally charge more for specific products or, instead of charging a percent tax, charge a dollar amount per ounce or pound wholesale only [8]. As with all things cannabis, revenue is an ever-changing facet.

Again, considering Colorado's revenue specifically, 0.85% of the state budget in Fiscal Year 2019 came from marijuana revenue. This equals $262 million of the $30.6 million total budget with the majority of this coming from retail marijuana taxes v. medical marijuana taxes [42].

Conclusion

As more and more states legalize the use of cannabis, use continues to increase. Cannabis use is harmful for the developing brain and there is hope that interventions targeting at risk populations, especially adolescents, can potentially decrease use. Older and medically ill patients are increasingly using cannabis without clear beneficial effect. Similarly, cannabis use is frequently comorbid with mental health diagnoses, especially other substance use diagnoses, though has not been found to be helpful in treating mental health conditions. Even with these negative effects, cannabis use is most clearly dangerous when a factor in car accidents. Despite use being legal to at least some degree in most states, drug trafficking of cannabis continues to be an increasing challenge in all states. And finally, the economic impact of cannabis legalization continues to evolve with the current cost/benefit ratio unknown (Highlights Box 1.1 and 1.2).

Highlights Box 1.1 Key Points for Patient Psychoeducation

- Cannabis laws continue to evolve in all U.S. states.
- Cannabis use is increasing in all states, regardless of degree of legalization.
- Cannabis use has not been found to be helpful for medical or mental health diagnoses.
- Crime relating to cannabis continues to increase despite increasing legalization.
- The economic impact of cannabis use is yet to be determined.

Highlights Box 1.2 Key Points in Treatment and Management

- Consider accidental cannabis exposures in young children and provide parents with anticipatory guidance regarding risks of parental use and importance of safe storage as with all poisons.
- Educate adolescents and pregnant and nursing women regarding negative impacts of cannabis use for the developing brain and counsel cessation.
- Assess for cannabis use at all visits and counsel patients on the risks of use and alternative treatment options for their stated concern.
- Counsel all patients against cannabis use and driving.

References

1. United Nations Office on Drugs and Crime. World drug report 2018 Vienna, Austria. 2018 [updated June 2018]. https://www.unodc.org/wdr2018/.
2. Carliner H, Mauro PM, Brown QL, Shmulewitz D, Rahim-Juwel R, Sarvet AL, et al. The widening gender gap in marijuana use prevalence in the U.S. during a period of economic change, 2002-2014. Drug Alcohol Depend. 2017;170:51–8.
3. Chandra S, Radwan MM, Majumdar CG, Church JC, Freeman TP, ElSohly MA. Correction to: new trends in cannabis potency in USA and Europe during the last decade (2008-2017). Eur Arch Psychiatry Clin Neurosci. 2019;269(8):997.
4. Onders B, Casavant MJ, Spiller HA, Chounthirath T, Smith GA. Marijuana exposure among children younger than six years in the United States. Clin Pediatr (Phila). 2016;55(5):428–36.
5. Azofeifa A, Mattson ME, Grant A. Monitoring marijuana use in the United States: challenges in an evolving environment. JAMA. 2016;316(17):1765–6.
6. Brown QL, Sarvet AL, Shmulewitz D, Martins SS, Wall MM, Hasin DS. Trends in marijuana use among pregnant and nonpregnant reproductive-aged women, 2002-2014. JAMA. 2017;317(2):207–9.
7. Han BH, Palamar JJ. Trends in cannabis use among older adults in the United States, 2015-2018. JAMA Intern Med. 2020;180(4):609–11.
8. Hartman M. Cannabis overview. Denver, CO: National Conference of State Legislatures; 2021 [updated March 31]. https://www.ncsl.org/research/civil-and-criminal-justice/marijuana-overview.aspx.
9. Hasin DS. US epidemiology of cannabis use and associated problems. Neuropsychopharmacology. 2018;43(1):195–212.
10. Compton MT, American Psychiatric Association. Marijuana and mental health, vol. xii. 1st ed. Arlington, VA: American Psychiatric Association Publishing; 2016, 243pp
11. Bonn-Miller MO, Boden MT, Bucossi MM, Babson KA. Self-reported cannabis use characteristics, patterns and helpfulness among medical cannabis users. Am J Drug Alcohol Abuse. 2014;40(1):23–30.
12. Reinarman C, Nunberg H, Lanthier F, Heddleston T. Who are medical marijuana patients? Population characteristics from nine California assessment clinics. J Psychoactive Drugs. 2011;43(2):128–35.
13. Pacula RL, MacCoun R, Reuter P, Chriqui J, Kilmer B, Harris K, et al. What does it mean to decriminalize marijuana? A cross-national empirical examination. Adv Health Econ Health Serv Res. 2005;16:347–69.
14. Whitehill JM, Harrington C, Lang CJ, Chary M, Bhutta WA, Burns MM. Incidence of pediatric cannabis exposure among children and teenagers aged 0 to 19 years before and after medical marijuana Legalization in Massachusetts. JAMA Netw Open. 2019;2(8):e199456.
15. Richards JR, Smith NE, Moulin AK. Unintentional cannabis ingestion in children: a systematic review. J Pediatr. 2017;190:142–52.
16. American Association of Poison Control Centers National Poison Data System. Cannabidiol (CBD). Arlington, VA; 2021. https://aapcc.org/CBD-Alert.
17. Shahzade C, Chun J, DeLisi LE, Manschreck TC. Patterns in adolescent cannabis use predict the onset and symptom structure of schizophrenia-spectrum disorder. Schizophr Res. 2018;197:539–43.
18. Gibbs M, Winsper C, Marwaha S, Gilbert E, Broome M, Singh SP. Cannabis use and mania symptoms: a systematic review and meta-analysis. J Affect Disord. 2015;171:39–47.
19. Navarrete F, Garcia-Gutierrez MS, Gasparyan A, Austrich-Olivares A, Femenia T, Manzanares J. Cannabis use in pregnant and breastfeeding women: behavioral and neurobiological consequences. Front Psych. 2020;11:586447.
20. Davis E, Lee T, Weber JT, Bugden S. Cannabis use in pregnancy and breastfeeding: the pharmacist's role. Can Pharm J (Ott). 2020;153(2):95–100.

21. Dai H, Richter KP. A national survey of marijuana use among US adults with medical conditions, 2016-2017. JAMA Netw Open. 2019;2(9):e1911936.
22. Calabria B, Degenhardt L, Hall W, Lynskey M. Does cannabis use increase the risk of death? Systematic review of epidemiological evidence on adverse effects of cannabis use. Drug Alcohol Rev. 2010;29(3):318–30.
23. Borges G, Bagge CL, Orozco R. A literature review and meta-analyses of cannabis use and suicidality. J Affect Disord. 2016;195:63–74.
24. San Nicolas AC, Lemos NP. Toxicology findings in cases of hanging in the City and County of San Francisco over the 3-year period from 2011 to 2013. Forensic Sci Int. 2015;255:146–55.
25. Drummer OH, Gerostamoulos D, Woodford NW. Cannabis as a cause of death: a review. Forensic Sci Int. 2019;298:298–306.
26. Asbridge M, Hayden JA, Cartwright JL. Acute cannabis consumption and motor vehicle collision risk: systematic review of observational studies and meta-analysis. BMJ. 2012;344:e536.
27. Li MC, Brady JE, DiMaggio CJ, Lusardi AR, Tzong KY, Li G. Marijuana use and motor vehicle crashes. Epidemiol Rev. 2012;34:65–72.
28. Liu C, Huang Y, Pressley JC. Restraint use and risky driving behaviors across drug types and drug and alcohol combinations for drivers involved in a fatal motor vehicle collision on U.S. roadways. Inj Epidemiol. 2016;3(1):9.
29. Hartman RL, Huestis MA. Cannabis effects on driving skills. Clin Chem. 2013;59(3):478–92.
30. Zhu H, Wu LT. Trends and correlates of cannabis-involved emergency department visits: 2004 to 2011. J Addict Med. 2016;10(6):429–36.
31. Gubatan J, Staller K, Barshop K, Kuo B. Cannabis abuse is increasing and associated with increased emergency department utilization in gastroenterology patients. Dig Dis Sci. 2016;61(7):1844–52.
32. Shelton SK, Mills E, Saben JL, Devivo M, Williamson K, Abbott D, et al. Why do patients come to the emergency department after using cannabis? Clin Toxicol (Phila). 2020;58(6):453–9.
33. Karila L, Roux P, Rolland B, Benyamina A, Reynaud M, Aubin HJ, et al. Acute and long-term effects of cannabis use: a review. Curr Pharm Des. 2014;20(25):4112–8.
34. Ecker AH, Lang B, Hogan J, Cucciare MA, Lindsay J. Cannabis use disorder among veterans: comorbidity and mental health treatment utilization. J Subst Abus Treat. 2020;109:46–9.
35. Budney AJ, Sofis MJ, Borodovsky JT. An update on cannabis use disorder with comment on the impact of policy related to therapeutic and recreational cannabis use. Eur Arch Psychiatry Clin Neurosci. 2019;269(1):73–86.
36. Lowe DJE, Sasiadek JD, Coles AS, George TP. Cannabis and mental illness: a review. Eur Arch Psychiatry Clin Neurosci. 2019;269(1):107–20.
37. Charilaou P, Agnihotri K, Garcia P, Badheka A, Frenia D, Yegneswaran B. Trends of cannabis use disorder in the inpatient: 2002 to 2011. Am J Med. 2017;130(6):678–87 e7.
38. Shi Y. Medical marijuana policies and hospitalizations related to marijuana and opioid pain reliever. Drug Alcohol Depend. 2017;173:144–50.
39. Jehle CC Jr, Nazir N, Bhavsar D. The rapidly increasing trend of cannabis use in burn injury. J Burn Care Res. 2015;36(1):e12–7.
40. Rai HS, Winder GS. Marijuana use and organ transplantation: a review and implications for clinical practice. Curr Psychiatry Rep. 2017;19(11):91.
41. United States Drug Enforcement Administration. 2020 national drug threat assessment. Washington, DC: United States Department of Justice; 2021. https://www.dea.gov/documents/2021/03/02/2020-national-drug-threat-assessment
42. The legalization of marijuana in Colorado: the impact, Vol 7. Rocky Mountain HIDTA Training and Information Center; 2020 [updated September]. https://www.thenmi.org/wp-content/uploads/2020/10/RMHIDTA-Marijuana-Report-2020-2.pdf.
43. Hughes L, Schaible L, Jimmerson K. Marijuana dispensaries and neighborhood crime and disorder in Denver, Colorado. Justice Quarterly. 2019;37:1–25.

44. Connealy N, Piza E, Hatten D. The criminogenic effect of marijuana dispensaries in Denver, Colorado: a microsynthetic control quasi-experiment and cost-benefit analysis. Justice Eval J. 2020;3(1):69–93.
45. Quest DIagnostics. Workforce drug testing positivity climbed to highest rate in 16 years, new quest diagnostics drug testing index™ analysis finds Secaucus, NJ, Quest Diagnostics; 2020 [updated August 25]. https://www.questdiagnostics.com/home/physicians/health-trends/drug-testing/.
46. Marijuana tax revenue in states that regulate marijuana for adult use. Washington, DC: Marijuana Policy Project; 2021. https://www.mpp.org/issues/legalization/marijuana-tax-revenue-states-regulate-marijuana-adult-use/.

Part I

Pharmacology of Cannabis

Clinical Pharmacology of Cannabinoids 2

Andrew Kluemper

Medical marijuana use in the United States has precipitously increased over the last two decades since California first approved medical use in 1996. It is frequently self-prescribed for a variety of indications ranging from chemotherapy-induced nausea and promotion of weight gain to post-traumatic stress disorder and generalized anxiety disorder. The indications and dispensing of medical marijuana are not regulated by the traditional processes that involve rigorous clinical trials and Food and Drug Administration (FDA) approval. State health departments are often tasked with determining what indications are approved. Patients can grow their own if they so wish, buy as much as they want, and use in whatever amount they see fit for that day. Loose marijuana contains no less than 50 distinct phytocannabinoids with unique activities and kinetics in the human body, making it extremely difficult to study each compound in a scientific fashion. Compounded with the fact that marijuana plants can range in the concentration and ratio of each cannabinoid, patients can experience vastly different effects from a similar ingestion of marijuana that make it even more problematic to determine which compound in which dose has what level of effect on the human body. Drug Enforcement Agency (DEA) scheduling has also historically created barriers to research, further compounding the knowledge gap. Patients turn to medical providers for information on medical marijuana; however, the medical education system only recently began discussing marijuana as a therapeutic drug and many physicians may not feel prepared to discuss marijuana [1]. As a result, patients turn to marijuana dispensary staff (colloquially known as "budtenders") for education about the product. Some states do require dispensaries to have a pharmacist on site who may have specialized marijuana education and can provide education, screen for drug interactions, and discuss potential adverse events. As of 2020, at least 33 states approved medical marijuana in some fashion with that number likely to continue to grow as time progresses. Some states

A. Kluemper (✉)
Pharmacy Department, University of Colorado Hospital, Aurora, CO, USA
e-mail: andrew.kluemper@uchealth.org

P. Riggs, T. Thant (eds.), *Cannabis in Psychiatric Practice*, Psychiatry Update 3,
https://doi.org/10.1007/978-3-031-04874-6_2

approved only CBD and regulate how much THC can be present in products in accordance with the 2018 Farm Bill which removed *Cannabis sativa* or "hemp" and other products with <0.3% THC content from the definition of marijuana, thus removing these products from controlled substance scheduling [2]. Unraveling the complexities of medical marijuana use and its potential benefits and risks starts with the endocannabinoid system, pharmacodynamics and pharmacokinetics of different cannabinoids, available dosage forms, adverse events, and drug interactions.

Endocannabinoid System Review [3–7]

Pharmacodynamics

The endocannabinoid (EC) system contains two main cannabinoid (CB) receptors—CB1 and CB2. In addition to these receptors, there are a number of postulated nonreceptor effects the endocannabinoid system is responsible for—ranging from immunomodulation to circulation.

CB receptors make up the majority of G-coupled protein receptors (GPCR) in the human brain. CB1 receptors are predominantly located in the central nervous system (CNS), but may also be found in peripheral organs—including the gastrointestinal tract and heart. CB2 receptors are largely located in the peripheral nervous system and immune system. CB1 receptors are thought to be the major receptor responsible for the psychoactive effects of marijuana.

CB1 receptors are highly concentrated in cognitive and emotional areas of the brain, namely the cerebral cortex and hippocampus. Activation causes downstream effects on acetylcholine, cAMP, GABA, glutamate, norepinephrine, serotonin, and dopamine, with resulting psychoactive effects. ECs also have a role in negative feedback systems. Presynaptic release of neurotransmitters triggers synthesis and release of ECs from postsynaptic cells. These ECs will bind to presynaptic CB receptors and inhibit neurotransmitter release via reduced influx of calcium, hyperpolarization, and decrease in the number of action potentials, and therefore decreasing frequency of neurotransmitter vesicle binding and release. ECs are metabolized by monoacylglycerol lipases (MAGL) and fatty acid amide hydrolase (FAAH) to inactive compounds. Development of MAGL and FAAH inhibitors (which would theoretically increase the half-life and clinical activity of ECs and reduce the production of inflammatory mediators) is ongoing (Fig. 2.1).

There are very few receptors present in the brainstem which correlates with marijuana's lack of cardiopulmonary toxicity, even at extreme doses [3]. Rat models have shown cannabinoids can inhibit the activation of serotonin subtype 3 receptors (the same receptors acted on by ondansetron), which fits with the antiemetic activity seen with cannabinoids. CB1 is activated by a number of cannabinoids, most notably delta-9-tetrahydrocannabinol (THC).

CB2 receptors are largely located on immune and other noncentral nervous system cells, but are also present in the central nervous system. CB2 activation does not lead to psychoactive effects, rather, it is thought that CB2 receptors are responsible

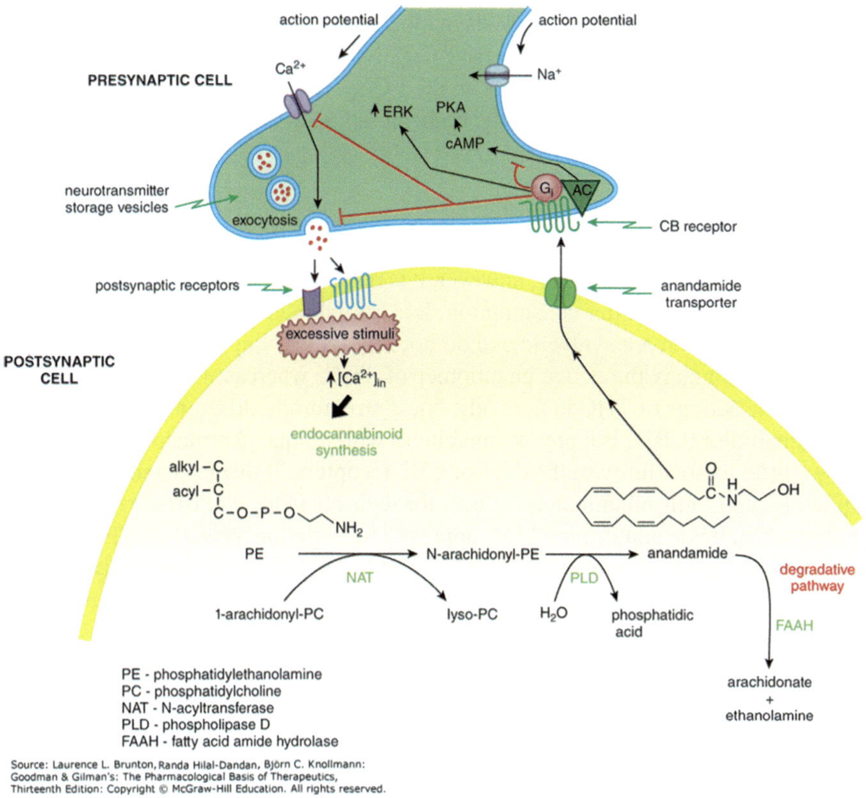

Fig. 2.1 Overview of cannabinoid neurotransmission in the central nervous system. Used with permission [8]

for immunomodulation, anti-inflammatory effects, and antineoplastic properties [5]. Development of pure CB2 modulators for immunomodulation has been attempted in the past; however, none have been successful as they have failed to eliminate CB1 activity and thus retain psychoactive properties. Cannabinoids can have various effects at CB2 receptors, including agonist and antagonist activities [3–7].

Cannabinoid Subtypes

There are three types of cannabinoids—endocannabinoids (cannabinoids our body makes), phytocannabinoids (exogenous cannabinoids found in plants), and synthetic cannabinoids (human-designed cannabinoids, generally only used recreationally).

Endocannabinoids (ECs)

Anandamide and 2-arachidonoylglycerol are the two most common ECs. Anandamide may have partial CB1 agonist activity, antagonist activity, and allosteric modulation depending on the concentration present. It has a lower affinity for the CB1 receptor than THC and 2 arachidonoylglycerol (which is a full agonist at CB receptors) [6, 9]. In addition to postsynaptic effects which modulate a variety of neurotransmitter releases, ECs also have negative feedback activity and bind to presynaptic neurons (see above section on the EC system for more information). ECs have a wide variety of activities in the body including effects on inflammation, pain, and the immune system.

Phytocannabinoids [10, 11]

THC is one of the most predominant phytocannabinoids present in marijuana. It has balanced CB1 and CB2 activity; however, it is responsible for most of the psychoactive effects that occur after consumption. It is available in two FDA-approved products, both of which are synthetic and do not rely on growing cannabis. Dronabinol (Marinol®) contains the active enantiomer of THC, whereas nabilone (Cesamet®) mimics the actions of THC in the body, but is structurally different.

Cannabidiol (CBD) is a phytocannabinoid with unique pharmacodynamics, as it shows little to no affinity to the CB1 or CB2 receptors. It displays antiemetic, antiepileptic, and anti-inflammatory effects through other mechanisms which are not fully known. It is available in an FDA-approved formulation (brand name Epidiolex®) for Lennox-Gastaut syndrome and Dravet syndrome [12]. It is commonly used for sleep and pain when purchased from medical dispensaries. CBD will be discussed in more detail in Chap. 3.

While not available in the United States, nabiximols (Sativex®) is an oromucosal spray made up of cannabis extracts. The primary components are equal ratios of THC and CBD; other cannabinoids are present in minor concentrations. It is approved for muscle spasticity related to multiple sclerosis in several countries in Europe and Asia. At the time of writing, clinical trials for United States approval are ongoing, and it is not FDA approved for use [13].

Patients may use the term "medical marijuana" to refer to high CBD content products with low THC or think that "medical marijuana" has little to no psychoactive properties. Some states, such as Indiana, have only approved CBD products and require that THC concentrations are below a certain threshold (0.3%) in accordance with the 2018 Farm Bill [2]; however, many states do not regulate cannabinoid content. It is important to clarify with patients if they are using predominantly CBD or THC products, what their usual product ratio is, what preparation is being used (concentrates, loose flower, dabs, etc.), and how they are administering (i.e., vaping, dabbing, smoking, oral, topical, etc.). It can be helpful to talk through information they receive from "budtenders" (people working at the dispensary who commonly make recommendations on which specific product/strain to use for specific indications—a largely unproven and unvalidated recommendation) to address potentially incorrect information provided.

Synthetic Cannabinoids [14]

Synthetic cannabinoids are generally used only recreationally. They are designed to have very high CB1 affinity [5]. After being synthesized in laboratories, they are usually sprayed onto plants and smoked. Consumer packaging often will state "not for human consumption" and will sometimes be marketed as potpourri to avoid legal consequences. There are many different molecules in this class and many different slang names, including "K2," "Spice," and "Black Mamba." [14] Just like other designer drugs, when a certain chemical compound in these products becomes illegal, manufacturers will alert the molecule very slightly to continue to sell legally. Patients using these drugs should be advised that they are even less regulated than medical marijuana, can have a variety of effects on users, and may have many negative medical and psychiatric effects. They should not be used for any medical purpose. Patients presenting with acute intoxication of these substances may present as agitated and delirious or obtunded and comatose. Reports of seizures, cerebral ischemia, myocardial infarction, acute kidney injury, and psychosis have all been reported in the literature. Mental status can vary widely during the course of their intoxication—some patients going from comatose to severely agitated within minutes.

Tolerance to Exogenous Cannabinoids [9, 15–18]

Tolerance to phytocannabinoids develops via downregulation of cannabinoid receptors over weeks to months of persistent use. Animal studies have showed that exposure to THC for 21 days leads to reduced CB receptor binding (i.e., desensitization) [9]. Reduction in CB receptor density and downstream coupling of GPCRs has also been observed in rodents with frequent exposure [15, 16]. Depending on the patient's desired effects, tolerance may lead to increased use as well as other adverse events, such as cannabinoid hyperemesis syndrome (discussed in Chap. 5.2). More potent CB agonists, including synthetic cannabinoids, have been shown to cause greater desensitization and receptor downregulation. Reversing tolerance to cannabinoids is variable but is generally on the order of weeks. A human study comparing chronic users (at least 2 years of regular use) with nonusers using radioactively labeled CB ligands showed 15% less binding of CB receptors in chronic users (due to receptor downregulation). Within chronic users, those with less binding reported more withdrawal symptoms. At both two and 28 days of observed abstinence, no difference in CB binding was detectable between chronic users and nonusers [17]. An earlier study by Ceccarini et al. showed 10–15% reduction in CB1 receptor binding after 4 days of abstinence in chronic users (using for an average of 10 years) when compared to nonusers. Together, these studies show CB receptor downregulation begins to reverse quickly, within days of cessation, and at 4 weeks, differences should be minimal, if present at all [18].

Dosage Forms

FDA-Approved Cannabinoids [10–12]

Dronabinol, nabilone, and cannabidiol are the three FDA-approved cannabinoid products currently available. Dronabinol and nabilone are controlled substances (schedule three and two, respectively). Cannabidiol was originally a schedule five controlled substance; however, in 2020, the DEA removed pharmaceutical cannabidiol from the list of controlled substances in response to data from animal and human studies that compared the abuse potential of cannabidiol, dronabinol, alprazolam, and placebo. Some states or institutions may still treat it as a controlled substance. All three of these products have quality and safety standards that are identical to other prescription drugs. While labeling of marijuana with cannabinoid concentrations and the dose present (especially in edibles) is becoming more widespread, the production of these products is less regulated than traditional prescription products. They may have other ingredients the patient (and dispensary) is not aware of. Cleanliness of these products is not guaranteed either. Reports of aspergillosis (a type of fungal pneumonia) after inhalation of contaminated marijuana have been published. Certain states, including Colorado, mandate either testing marijuana products for contaminants such as bacteria and mold, or labeling that it has not been tested for contaminants.

Dronabinol (Marinol®) [10] is indicated for anorexia associated with weight loss in adult patients with acquired immunodeficiency syndrome (AIDS) and for nausea and vomiting associated with chemotherapy in adult patients who failed conventional antiemetics. It is synthetic THC with similar pharmacologic activity.

Nabilone (Cesamet®) [11] is another THC analog with FDA indications for the treatment of nausea and vomiting associated with chemotherapy in patients who have failed to adequately respond to conventional antiemetics. It is not indicated for AIDS-related anorexia and weight loss. Like dronabinol, it has similar pharmacologic activity to THC and carries the same psychoactive properties.

Cannabinol (Epidiolex®) [12] is made by purifying cannabinoid extracts from cannabis grown in the United Kingdom. It is indicated for seizures associated with Lennox-Gastaut syndrome, Dravet syndrome, or tuberous sclerosis complex in patients one year of age or older. Clinical trials, as expected, showed very little clinical psychoactive properties outside of somnolence.

In addition to the three FDA-approved formulations, marijuana is available in a wide variety of dosage forms, including loose plant (mainly used for smoking), concentrated oils used for vaping or "dabbing," oral and sublingual products, topical creams, and even suppositories for menstrual cramping. Use of noninhalation dosage forms has risen significantly with legalization of medical and recreational marijuana. While some states have only legalized medical marijuana and some states do regulate THC and CBD ratios in products, for the most part, the products themselves can be dispensed as either recreational or medical. That is, there is nothing special about the medical marijuana product itself, outside of the fact that a prescription or physician order is required, different age limits may exist, and the tax structures are different.

Patients should be advised that smoking marijuana (i.e., burning of loose plant/flower) can still produce hydrocarbons that can be carcinogenic. For this reason, I generally recommend that patients using marijuana for medical reasons use edible or topical products.

Concentrations of THC present in marijuana have continually increased over the past 3 decades. In 2014, a study by the DEA showed that THC concentrations had almost tripled since 1995, largely attributed to the ability of growers to crossbreed hybrids of different strains of the *Cannabis* plant itself to increase THC and CBD concentrations and alter ratios of which phytocannabinoids are present [19]. Concentrates (i.e., butane hash oil, hash oil, dabs) are also increasing in popularity and have significant health implications. These products are highly concentrated THC products, with upwards of 80–90% THC content versus 15–30% seen in flower form. Patients can become extremely intoxicated very quickly and usually only need one or two inhalations. These products, because of their high concentration and fast onset, cause intense nervous system effects immediately, rather than a slower progression seen with smoking flower or using edibles. Patients who use concentrates may experience psychosis, hallucinations, agitation, paranoia, and cardiac adverse effects including palpitations. They may also become tolerant more quickly and experience more severe withdrawal effects. There are risks with certain dabbing devices, including burns. Production of concentrates can also be risky since a large amount of heat and combustible chemicals are needed. Like smoking, inhaled concentrates should not be recommended for medical use.

Oral dosage forms are commonly used in both medical and recreational settings. They lack the quick onset seen with inhalation and may result in fewer adverse psychiatric events. One of the largest risks associated with oral dosage forms is delayed onset. With inhalation, the effect is seen within minutes and the user can titrate their own dose as they see fit. With oral ingestion, patients may not see the effects for up to 3–4 h [20], so they might consume more before the first product has fully absorbed and consequently, find themselves more intoxicated and for a longer time than they hoped. This has become a public health issue as it relates to driving as a patient may consume an edible product, feel fine 1–2 h later, drive, and then become more and more intoxicated and sedated while driving.

Topical products, such as oils and lotions, are becoming more and more common. These products usually contain CBD only; however, THC products are also available. National brands such as Burt's Bees have started producing CBD-infused lotions marketed to improve skin hydration and moisturization. Most dispensaries market these products for pain, inflammation, and even psoriasis and eczema. Systemic absorption of these products is minimal and few people will report clinically relevant psychoactive effects, especially compared to inhalation. Transdermal THC patches are also available, and these products generally have higher systemic absorption and psychoactive properties.

Pharmacokinetics [3, 5–7, 9, 20]

Absorption

Absorption is route dependent. Patients should be advised that smoking marijuana products leads to rapid absorption and clinical effects within minutes, while edible products can take up to 3–4 h to have their peak effect [20]. Oral ingestion is subject to first pass metabolism in the liver which reduces the effective dose compared to inhalation. For example, dronabinol only has 10% bioavailability. This is in line with data on other oral cannabinoids of approximately 10–30% bioavailability. The figure below shows this difference in peak concentration and total absorption of oral vs. inhaled. Ingestion of oral cannabinoids with other food may increase the maximum concentration [11]. Topical products have very low bioavailability and generally do not reach the bloodstream in clinically significant amounts.

Distribution

The majority of cannabinoids, including THC and the metabolites 11-hydroxy THC (11-OH-THC) and 11-nor-9-carboxy-THC (THC-COOH), are very lipophilic compounds and readily distribute into the brain and adipose tissue. THC has an initial volume of distribution of 2.5–3.5 L/kg (i.e., around 210 L for a 70 kg patient), with chronic users displaying higher volumes of distribution of up to 100 times this [5], or about 21,000 L for a 70 kg patient—an incredibly high value which suggests extensive adipose tissue deposits. Some data suggests that CBD has a volume of distribution of 30 L/kg, or ten times that of THC. The clinical trials for cannabidiol (Epidiolex®) showed volumes of up to 42,000 L after only 7 days of use [12]. Distribution models with up to 6 compartments have been suggested, but most literature agrees that at least 2 phases exist [5]. Phase 1 involves distribution mainly with the plasma volume and is highly protein bound. This phase also distributes THC to highly vascularized tissues, such as the heart, lungs, and brain. Phase 2 involves distribution of THC and metabolites (inactive and active) to adipose tissue and less vascularized tissues. Chronic users redistribute inactive metabolites from adipose into blood and urine which is the underlying reason for positive urine drug screens weeks after last use and prolonged half-lives of different compounds. Cannabinoids cross the placenta easily and are also found in breastmilk. The relative infant dose possible during breastfeeding can be variable dependent on the mother's use patterns. Epidiolex® trials in animals showed increased risk of developmental toxicity. Cannabinoid use during pregnancy or breastfeeding is not recommended.

Metabolism

In addition to first pass metabolism, THC and CBD are hepatically metabolized via cytochrome P450 enzymes, namely 2C9 and 3A4. THC has some notable metabolites, both active and inactive. THC-COOH is a nonpsychotropic metabolite of THC that has anti-inflammatory properties. It has a half-life of 5–7 days. 11-OH-THC is a psychoactive metabolite with a half-life of 12–36 h. It has a similar kinetic profile to THC.

In addition to being metabolized by the P450 enzyme system, cannabinoids can inhibit these enzymes which further complicates their clinical presentation, clearance, and interactions with medications. In addition to cannabinoid effects, hydrocarbons produced during smoking will induce CYP1A2 which is responsible for the metabolism of a number of psychiatric medications, including clozapine, olanzapine, fluvoxamine, and duloxetine. Commonly used drug-drug interaction tools are generally not built to include interactions with marijuana; however, some drug information resources can incorporate marijuana interactions and as more research is published, these interaction tools should improve. Drug interactions will be discussed more in the next section.

Elimination

Cannabinoids and their metabolites eventually undergo glucuronidation and are eliminated in the urine and feces. As previously discussed, this process can be quite prolonged due to the highly lipophilic nature of cannabinoids that partition in adipose tissue and slowly equilibrate with the serum. Some chronic users may have detectable blood and urine concentrations up to 46 days from last use. Naïve users will have less adipose stores, shorter half-lives, and thus, will only test positive for 1–2 weeks after last use. The clinical trials for cannabidiol (Epidiolex®) showed elimination half-lives of 56–61 h after 7 days of administration in healthy volunteers. This is in line with studies evaluating THC use and a resulting half-life of up to 12 days in chronic users and as little as 2 h in naïve users, although it is difficult to compare these as serum THC half-life does not necessarily equal elimination half-life. THC-COOH is the primary urinary metabolite with a half-life of 5–7 days and causes a positive urine drug screen.

This figure below (used with permission from Goldfrank's Toxicologic Emergencies) shows the time course of THC and its metabolites. As you can see, chronic administration results in accumulation of THC-COOH (major nonpsychoactive metabolite). Oral administration results in a delayed peak of metabolites with higher concentrations versus smoking thanks to the first pass effect on THC, which shows relatively low concentrations relative to peaks seen with inhalation.

Figure 74-3, Goldfrank's Toxicologic Emergencies, 11e [21].

Estimated relative time course of delta-9-tetrahydrocannabinol (THC) and its major metabolite in the urine based on the route of exposure (Fig. 2.2).

Future drug tests may be able to incorporate ratio of metabolites to CBD and THC to determine when a patient last used. This is notably an issue in law enforcement where driving under the influence of marijuana is very subjective compared to alcohol use where clinical effects correlate well with blood alcohol levels.

Drug-Drug Interactions [5, 10–12, 22–25]

As previously discussed, CBD and THC have a variety of effects on CYP450 metabolism and effect a number of common enzymes responsible for drug metabolism. The purpose of this section will not be to detail every possible drug interaction. For patient-specific drug interactions, consultation with a pharmacist is recommended. Several drug databases, including Lexi-Comp®, have the ability to enter "marijuana" as a drug to screen for pharmaceutical drug interactions. This will

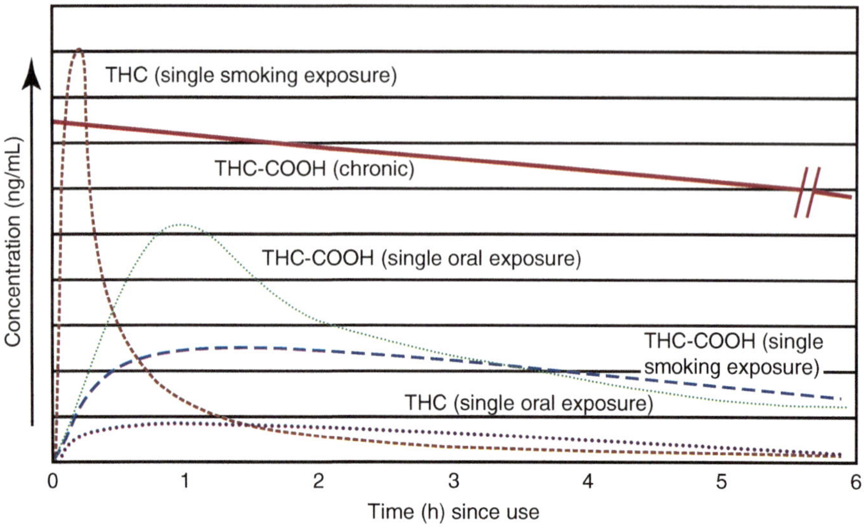

Source: L.S. Nelson, M.A. Howland, N.A. Lewin, S.W. Smith, L.R. Goldfrank
R.S. Hoffman: Goldfrank's Tosicologic Emergencies, Eleventh Edition

Fig. 2.2 Estimated relative time course of delta-9-tetrahydrocannabinol (THC) and its major metabolite in the urine based on the route of exposure. Used with permission

often group all cannabinoid containing products into one syntax, but one should evaluate this closely, especially if a patient is on high-risk medications or using pure CBD products (in which case "cannabidiol" should be entered as well). Some of this information relies on the FDA-approved package insert for pharmaceutical cannabinoids. Because of this grouping, it is possible for an interaction to alert when it actually does not exist based on the specific product being used. Route of administration also may further compound this issue. For this reason, consultation with a pharmacist is recommended, especially with high-risk interactions such as immunosuppressants, anticoagulants, antiepileptic drugs, cardiac medications, antiretrovirals, and many others.

Antidepressants go through a variety of CYP enzymes. For example, citalopram is metabolized by 2C19 and 2D6 to a certain extent. CBD's inhibition of both of these enzymes may increase the patient's concentrations of citalopram and cause adverse events (including serotonin syndrome) with a possible need for dose decreases. Venlafaxine has minor metabolism to active metabolites through 2C19, 2C9, 2D6, and 3A4. Use of CBD in a patient on venlafaxine may cause a reduction in active metabolites (desvenlafaxine) and high venlafaxine concentrations. Since venlafaxine and desvenlafaxine have different serotonin and norepinephrine activities at different doses, this change in activity at different receptors could cause decreased efficacy or increased side effects, and the patient should be counseled on this potential interaction.

If a patient is electing to begin using medical marijuana, it is important to screen their current medication list for possible new interactions and discuss these with the patient. This is yet another reason that providers should ask patients about the cannabinoid content and makeup of the products they are using.

CYP450 Properties of THC and CBD [5, 9, 25]

Enzyme	THC	CBD
3A4	Substrate	Substrate, inhibitor
2C9	Major substrate, weak inhibitor	Substrate, inhibitor
2C19	Substrate	Substrate, inhibitor
2D6	n/a	Substrate, inhibitor
1A2	Induced by smoking	Induced by smoking

Pharmacodynamic interactions exist as well and should be considered, especially in elderly patients or those using other psychoactive prescription or recreational drugs. Marijuana can cause additive sedation with other CNS depressants such as alcohol or benzodiazepines. Anticholinergic medications may cause even more profound dry mouth, red eyes, and other effects.

Drug interactions can differ based on the route of administration as well. Inhaled marijuana will be more susceptible to drug interactions due to CYP1A2 induction (responsible for clozapine and olanzapine metabolism) caused by the burning of hydrocarbons. Topical preparations may have few drug interactions due to low systemic absorption.

Adverse Events

Adverse events from marijuana use are common and quite variable. Psychiatric adverse events will largely be discussed later in this book, but acute psychiatric events including psychosis, paranoia, and anxiety are all possible, especially with synthetic cannabinoids and high potency marijuana concentrates. Medical adverse events can range from tachycardia, hypertension, and dry mouth to stupor, coma, ataxia, bradycardia, and hypotension. Medical adverse events are becoming more common with increased ED visits reported in Colorado by Monte et al. since legalization [26]. Toxic ingestions of edible marijuana products by children have increased numerically every year since legalization [27]. Some states now have more restrictions on edible products. Colorado, for example, now requires a large symbol on all edible products, requires each serving (10 mg of THC) of product to be individually packaged and labeled, and no longer allows the use of words such as "candy" or "gummy" on the packaging to help deter children from thinking it is only candy. Additionally, products must now have a potency statement [28].

Drug and Genetic Testing

Drug Testing

THC is one of the "federal five" drugs that is on routine employment drug screens (the other four being amphetamines, opiates, phencyclidine, and cocaine). Even as more states adopt medical and recreational marijuana, individual organizations can still elect to terminate employment based on failing this drug screen.

Urine drug screens (UDS) utilize enzyme-linked immunosorbent assays (ELISA) to detect drug in the urine. Antibodies in the test bind antigens (drugs and metabolites) in the urine. Different tests have different cutoffs for resulting as positive, but most facilities use the federal workplace cutoffs (50 mcg/mL). These screening tests are prone to false positives and false negatives, but they are relatively fast and inexpensive compared to gas chromatography and mass spectrometry (GC/MS) tests which isolate and identify specific molecules in the urine. GC/MS tests are used for confirmation testing and in detailed drug testing since many opioids and benzodiazepines have different structures, making it difficult to develop a single antibody that would bind all drugs in that class. Lastly, most cannabinoid UDSs do not report urine concentrations. Because of the wide variability in urine dilution, specific gravity, metabolism, and timing of last dose, any UDS that provides urinary concentrations does not necessarily mean the patient is clinically intoxicated.

Cannabinoid ELISA UDSs generally use a THC antibody to detect THC and the major metabolites (11-OH-THC and THC-COOH). THC-COOH's long half-life of 5–7 days and lack of psychoactive properties are the reason chronic marijuana users can have a positive UDS up to 30 days from their last use and display no clinical signs of intoxication.

Secondhand smoke should not trigger a positive UDS [29–32]. A recent study in 2015 by Cone et al. exposed patients to secondhand marijuana smoke in small rooms without ventilation for prolonged periods of 60 min each. They found only one subject tested positive at the federal cutoff (50 mcg/mL) 6 h after session 2 (total time of 2 h of exposure to secondhand smoke in a sealed room). At the 8-h mark, the subject fell below the federal cutoff. They concluded that positive UDS results from secondhand smoke were possible, but only under extreme conditions of a sealed room without ventilation and prolonged duration of exposure with obvious knowledge by the subjects that others in the room were consuming marijuana, and only if the patient was tested in the 6–8 h after exposure [29].

Summary

- THC and CBD are the two main phytocannabinoids present in marijuana. THC acts primarily as a CB1/2 receptor agonist. THC is responsible for psychoactive properties of marijuana.
- Medical marijuana comes in a variety of unregulated forms with variable contents and cannabinoids ratios. Providers should discuss which formulation a

patient is using, the route of administration, what the usual THC:CBD ratio is, how frequently they use, why they use, and what adverse effects they notice from use. Providers should educate patients about the potential adverse effects of marijuana if a patient is considering using medical marijuana for a specific condition.
- Providers should not hesitate to discuss and educate patients on marijuana use, as patients receive information from many sources of varying credibility.
- Recently, especially among recreational marijuana, THC content of loose marijuana has been increasing.
- When using marijuana medically, oral or topical use is preferred due to the known carcinogenic risk associated with hydrocarbons produced during smoking or burning marijuana and a lower risk of adverse psychiatric effects, including acute psychosis.
- Both pharmacokinetic and pharmacodynamic drug interactions can be an issue with marijuana use, and THC and CBD can have different effects on metabolism of other drugs. For patients on high-risk medications (including but not limited to immunosuppressants, anticoagulants, and antiepileptic drugs), consultation with a pharmacist is recommended.
- Chronic use can result in urine drug tests being positive for up to 30 days after cessation. Secondhand smoke will not cause a positive urine drug test.

References

1. Evanoff AB, Quan T, Dufault C, Awad M, Bierut LJ. Physicians-in-training are not prepared to prescribe medical marijuana. Drug Alcohol Depend. 2017;180:151–5.
2. Agricultural Improvement Act of 2018.HB2. 115th Congress. 2018.
3. Lapoint JM. Chapter 74: Cannabinoids. In: Nelson LS, Howland M, Lewin NA, Smith SW, Goldfrank LR, Hoffman RS, editors. Goldfrank's toxicologic emergencies, 11e. New York: McGraw-Hill.
4. Turcotte C, Blanchet MR, Laviolette M, Flamand N. The CB2 receptor and its role as a regulator of inflammation. Cell Mol Life Sci. 2016 Dec;73:4449–70.
5. Grotenhermen F. Pharmacokinetics and pharmacodynamics of cannabinoids. Clin Pharmacokinet. 2003;42:327–60.
6. Vanderah TW. Cannabinoid drugs. In: Katzung BG, Vanderah TW, editors. Basic & clinical pharmacology, 15e. New York: McGraw-Hill.
7. Free R, Clark J, Amara S, Sibley DR. Neurotransmission in the central nervous system. In: Brunton LL, Hilal-Dandan R, Knollmann BC, editors. Goodman & Gilman's: the pharmacological basis of therapeutics, 13e. New York: McGraw-Hill.
8. Free R, Clark J, Amara S, Sibley DR. Neurotransmission in the central nervous system. In: Brunton LL, Hilal-Dandan R, Knollmann BC, editors. Goodman & Gilman's: the pharmacological basis of therapeutics, 13e. New York: McGraw-Hill; Figure 14-17, Anandamide synthesis and signaling in the CNS.
9. Pertwee RG. The diverse CB1 and CB2 receptor pharmacology of three plant cannabinoids: delta9-tetrahydrocannabinol, cannabidiol and delta9-tetrahydrocannabivarin. Br J Pharmacol. 2008;153:199–215.
10. Marinol [package insert]. Parsippany, NJ: ThePharmaNetwork; 2019.
11. Cesamet [package insert]. Bridgewater, NJ: Bausch Health; 2020.
12. Epidiolex [package insert]. Carlsbad, CA: Greenwich Biosciences; 2020.
13. GW Pharmaceuticals. Sativex®. https://www.gwpharm.com/healthcare-professionals/sativex. Accessed 1 June 2021.

14. National Institute on Drug Abuse. Synthetic cannabinoid DrugFacts. https://www.drugabuse.gov/publications/drugfacts/synthetic-cannabinoids-k2spice. Accessed 27 April 2021.
15. Sim-Selley LJ, Martin BR. Effect of chronic administration of R-(+)-[2,3-Dihydro-5-methyl-3-[(morpholinyl)methyl]pyrrolo[1,2,3-de]-1,4-benzoxazinyl]-(1-naphthalenyl)methanone mesylate (WIN55,212-2) or delta(9)-tetrahydrocannabinol on cannabinoid receptor adaptation in mice. J Pharmacol Exp Ther. 2002;303:36–44.
16. Breivogel CS, Griffin G, Di Marzo V, Martin BR. Evidence for a new G protein-coupled cannabinoid receptor in mouse brain. Mol Pharmacol. 2001;60:155–63.
17. D'Souza DC, Cortes-Briones JA, Ranganathan M, Thurnauer H, Creatura G, Surti T, Planeta B, Neumeister A, Pittman B, Normandin MD, Kapinos M, Ropchan J, Huang Y, Carson RE, Skosnik PD. Rapid changes in cannabinoid 1 receptor availability in cannabis-dependent male subjects after abstinence from cannabis. Biol Psychiatry Cogn Neurosci Neuroimaging. 2016;1:60–7.
18. Ceccarini J, Kuepper R, Kemels D, van Os J, Henquet C, Van Laere K. [18F]MK-9470 PET measurement of cannabinoid CB1 receptor availability in chronic cannabis users. Addict Biol. 2015;20:357–67.
19. ElSohly MA, Mehmedic Z, Foster S, Gon C, Chandra S, Church JC. Changes in cannabis potency over the last 2 decades (1995-2014): analysis of current data in the United States. Biol Psychiatry. 2016;79:613–9.
20. Vandrey R, Herrmann ES, Mitchell JM, Bigelow GE, Flegel R, LoDico C, Cone EJ. Pharmacokinetic profile of oral cannabis in humans: blood and Oral fluid disposition and relation to pharmacodynamic outcomes. J Anal Toxicol. 2017;41:83–99.
21. Lapoint JM. Chapter 74: Cannabinoids. In: Nelson LS, Howland M, Lewin NA, Smith SW, Goldfrank LR, Hoffman RS, editors. Goldfrank's toxicologic emergencies, 11e. New York: McGraw-Hill; Figure 74-3, Estimated relative time course of delta-9-tetrahydrocannabinol (THC) and its major metabolite in the urine based on the route of exposure.
22. Cannabidiol, Marijuana. Interactions. Lexicomp. Riverwoods, IL:Wolters Kluwer Health, Inc. Accessed 24 August 2016. http://online.lexi.com
23. Citalopram. Lexi-Drugs. Lexicomp. Riverwoods, IL:Wolters Kluwer Health, Inc. Accessed 1 June 2021. http://online.lexi.com
24. Venlafaxine. Lexi-Drugs. Lexicomp. Riverwoods, IL:Wolters Kluwer Health, Inc. Accessed 1 June 2021. http://online.lexi.com
25. Qian Y, Gurley BJ, Markowitz JS. The potential for pharmacokinetic interactions between cannabis products and conventional medications. J Clin Psychopharmacol. 2019;39:462–71.
26. Monte AA, Shelton SK, Mills E, Saben J, Hopkinson A, Sonn B, Devivo M, Chang T, Fox J, Brevik C, Williamson K, Abbott D. Acute illness associated with cannabis use, by route of exposure: an observational study. Ann Intern Med. 2019;170:531–7.
27. Wang GS, Le Lait MC, Deakyne SJ, Bronstein AC, Bajaj L, Roosevelt G. Unintentional Pediatric Exposures to Marijuana in Colorado, 2009-2015. JAMA Pediatr. 2016;170:e160971.
28. Colorado Department of Public Health and Environment. New Colorado rules make marijuana packaging safer for adults, less appealing to children. 2016. https://www.colorado.gov/pacific/marijuana/news/new-colorado-rules-make-marijuana-packaging-safer-adults-less-appealing-children. Accessed 28 April 2021.
29. Cone EJ, Bigelow GE, Herrmann ES, et al. Non-smoker exposure to secondhand cannabis smoke, I: urine screening and confirmation results. J Anal Toxicol. 2015;39:1–12.
30. Mulé SJ, Lomax P, Gross SJ. Active and realistic passive marijuana exposure tested by three immunoassays and GC/MS in urine. J Anal Toxicol. 1988;12:113–6.
31. Perez-Reyes M, Di Guiseppi S, Mason AP, Davis KH. Passive inhalation of marihuana smoke and urinary excretion of cannabinoids. Clin Pharmacol Ther. 1983;34:36–41.
32. Cone EJ, Johnson RE, Darwin WD, et al. Passive inhalation of marijuana smoke: urinalysis and room air levels of delta-9- tetrahydrocannabinol. J Anal Toxicol. 1987;11:89–96.

Cannabidiol: Overview, Complexities, and Opportunities for Behavioral Health

3

Susan R.B. Weiss and Katia Delrahim Howlett

What Is Cannabidiol (CBD)?

The cannabis plant has been recognized for thousands of years for its medicinal and recreational properties. This includes cannabidiol (CBD)-rich varieties; for instance, Queen Victoria in the nineteenth century reportedly treated her menstrual cramps using a variety of cannabis thought to be high in CBD. However, the specific components of the cannabis plant responsible for its therapeutic and psychoactive effects were unknown until the mid-twentieth century. CBD was first isolated from the cannabis plant in the early 1940s [1]; but it was not until 1963 that Raphael Mechoulam (known as the "Father of Cannabis Research") identified its full molecular structure; a year later, he described the structure of delta-9-tetrahydrocannabinol (THC) [2]. These developments were foundational for understanding the actions of cannabinoids and how they might be used in a therapeutic context. It was also Mechoulam who identified THC as the main component of the plant responsible for its psychotropic effects and noted that CBD lacked those properties.

Although much of the research that followed focused on THC, which led to the seminal discovery of the endocannabinoid system (see Chaps. 2 and 4), there were also anecdotal reports of potential antiepileptic effects of cannabis. Early studies conducted in mice and rats in the 1970s reported that CBD was effective in several seizure models [e.g., focal seizure models, maximal electroshock (MES) generalized seizures, electrically kindled limbic seizures] [3, 4]. Mechoulam and his team

The views and opinions expressed in this chapter are those of the authors only and do not necessarily represent the views, official policy, or position of the U.S. Department of Health and Human Services or any of its affiliated institutions or agencies.

S. R.B. Weiss (✉) · K. Delrahim Howlett
Division of Extramural Research, National Institutes of Health, National Institute on Drug Abuse, Bethesda, MD, USA
e-mail: sweiss@nida.nih.gov

P. Riggs, T. Thant (eds.), *Cannabis in Psychiatric Practice*, Psychiatry Update 3,
https://doi.org/10.1007/978-3-031-04874-6_3

conducted the first clinical trial of CBD for epilepsy in 1980. They administered daily doses of 300 mg of CBD to a small number of patients (*N* = 8) with epilepsy whose seizures were not controlled by their current medications [5]. Over a 4-month period, half of the patients became seizure free, and 3 of the remaining 4 showed a decrease in the frequency of their seizures. All tolerated the CBD well with few side effects. This was an important finding that would go relatively unnoticed for many years until CBD was once again brought to the public's attention by Sanjay Gupta in a 2014 CNN Special Report, "Weed" [6]. Dr. Gupta focused on a high-CBD strain of cannabis named Charlotte's Web™, initially grown by the Stanley brothers in Colorado for a child named Charlotte Figi who was being successfully treated for a severe form of epilepsy that was not controlled by anticonvulsant medications. Also, beginning in 2014, a series of studies using a purified cannabis extract that contained more than 99% CBD (Epidiolex®, GW Pharmaceuticals, Cambridge, UK) was being tested for its efficacy for severe pediatric-onset epilepsies.

Subsequently, CBD became widely known for a burgeoning set of potential therapeutic properties and for its relatively low toxicity. Although some of its proposed applications have some support in preclinical (in vitro or in vivo) research and "biological plausibility," most of the reported clinical successes are based on anecdote. The exceptions are the antiepileptic properties and, to a lesser degree, its antianxiety effects, which have been demonstrated in multiple human laboratory studies and a few clinical trials [7]. Though the promise of potential therapeutic applications for CBD remains strong, the current marketing and sales of CBD products are mostly without scientific substantiation.

Is CBD Legal?

The U.S. legal and regulatory framework for CBD is complex and differences among the state and federal laws add to confusion around its current legal status. The enactment of H.R.2 - Agriculture Improvement Act of 2018 (commonly known as the Farm Bill) amended the Controlled Substances Act (21 U.S.C. 802(16)) to distinguish "hemp" from "marijuana" based on the delta-9 THC content of the plant *Cannabis sativa*, and it modified the definition of tetrahydrocannabinols (category of cannabinoids either found in Cannabis or synthetically created in a lab) to exclude the compounds found in hemp (SEC. 12619) [8]. The bill defines hemp as varieties of cannabis (including the seeds and all derivatives, extracts, cannabinoids, isomers, acids, salts, and salts of isomers) with a delta-9 THC concentration of less than 0.3% (dry weight). In 2020, the Drug Enforcement Administration (DEA) (the federal agency that enforces the Controlled Substances Act) published an interim final rule to establish that the DEA considers the following as Schedule I controlled substances: (1) derivatives of hemp containing delta-9 THC in excess of 0.3%, and (2) all synthetic cannabinoids [9]. Therefore, while the Farm Bill removed hemp-derived CBD from the jurisdiction of the DEA, the interim final rule has introduced another layer of complexity for synthetic versions of CBD.

The Farm Bill preserved the authority of the Food and Drug Administration (FDA) to regulate products containing cannabis-derived compounds like any other food and drug products, regardless of whether they come from marijuana or hemp. In 2018, the FDA approved Epidiolex®, which contains a marijuana derived, purified form of CBD for treating seizures associated with Dravet or Lennox-Gastaut syndrome; and 2 years later, it approved the drug for a new indication (seizures associated with Tuberous Sclerosis), concluding that the product is safe and effective for its intended use [10]. In addition, the Drug Enforcement Agency (DEA) descheduled Epidiolex® from Schedule V, reserved for substances with low abuse liability, to a noncontrolled substance. However, neither the FDA approval nor the DEA reclassification extend to other CBD formulations (or other medical indications). Further, the Federal Drug and Cosmetic Act (FD&C Act) *prohibits* an active ingredient in an approved drug product (or one that was the subject of substantial clinical investigations, instituted or established, and such investigations were made public) from being added to human or animal foods; it also excludes products containing the active ingredient from the definition of a dietary supplement. CBD is therefore an unapproved food additive, and its use in human or animal food violates the FD&C Act as does its marketing or sales as a dietary supplement.

Because the Farm Bill preserved the FDA's regulatory authority over hemp products, a determination will need to be made on how best to implement and enforce regulations. The FDA is actively soliciting real world data to understand the safety of these products and inform subsequent regulatory actions. They have issued warning letters to manufacturers making false claims about CBD products for treating serious diseases (e.g., cancer) and they continue to perform analyses of CBD products for contaminants and labeling accuracy. Regardless of whether the product is derived from hemp or marijuana, clinical research to evaluate the safety and efficacy of CBD, as with any pharmaceutical formulation, requires FDA review and approval. This ensures consistency in product dosing and safety in growing conditions and other aspects of manufacturing related to the CBD formulation.

Additionally, each state handles CBD differently, and state regulations are not always aligned with federal regulations [11]. Even prior to the passage of the Farm Bill, 11 states had passed laws allowing the use of "low THC, high cannabidiol (CBD)" products for limited medical use (most often, seizure disorders). The amount of THC specified in these laws varied; but most products would not meet the legal definition of hemp. Most of these laws were passed prior to the FDA approval of Epidiolex®.

Thus, there are multiple and conflicting laws and regulations concerning high-CBD products. The recent proliferation of CBD products in the U.S. market does not have adequate oversight, and products often lack proper labeling of constituents, and/or make unsubstantiated health claims. An industry now estimated at more than a billion dollars has been able to flourish unregulated.

How Does CBD Work?

CBD is a potent antioxidant and anti-inflammatory drug, which could impart multiple beneficial effects on health. The numerous molecular targets and signaling pathways that CBD acts on have been reviewed elsewhere [12–15]. Determining which are most important for the large variety of conditions that CBD is purported to treat has proven difficult. Here, we will focus on a small subset of targets that have received considerable attention and have been linked to potential therapeutic effects of CBD, mostly assessed in preclinical studies.

Endocannabinoid System: In the late 1980 and 1990s, prompted by the identification and structural characterization of THC and other cannabinoids, researchers discovered a previously unknown signaling system in the brain and the body comprising CB1 and CB2 receptors, the endogenous ligands anandamide (N-arachidonoylethanolamine; AEA) and 2-Arachidonoylglycerol (2-AG), and the enzymes responsible for their synthesis and breakdown. Notably, the CB1 and CB2 receptors do not appear to play a major role in CBD's in vivo effects at the doses or concentrations necessary to produce pharmacological effects. However, CBD may attenuate some of the effects of THC by acting as a negative allosteric regulator of the CB1 receptor, biasing the receptor against THC's partial-agonist actions. CBD also increases the levels of the endogenous cannabinoid anandamide, possibly through blockade of the enzyme responsible for anandamide breakdown (fatty acid amide hydrolase or FAAH); however, this effect may be restricted to the rodent form of FAAH and not its human analog [16, 17].

Interestingly, in human studies, both antagonistic and synergistic actions have been reported for THC and CBD, which likely depend on dose, route of administration, effect being measured, timing and chronicity of administration, plant product or isolated cannabinoids, and other factors. CBD has been shown to moderate the psychotomimetic effects of THC. This is a significant issue because the breeding of cannabis for high levels of THC (to increase the euphoric effects) also reduces CBD to trace amounts. This change in ratio of the two main cannabinoids has been postulated as one reason for the increases in psychotic symptoms as well as psychotic illness in cannabis users reported in some studies [18, 19]. Consistent with this idea, users of products with greater levels of CBD (based on hair or saliva samples) showed fewer cognitive deficits, and in some studies reduced paranoia symptoms [20, 21].

Human laboratory studies have thus far failed to show consistent effects of CBD administration on responses to THC [22]; nevertheless, it has been suggested that cannabis plants bred to contain higher levels of CBD could be a harm-reduction strategy to address some of THCs adverse effects [23]. In contrast, some of the potential therapeutic effects of CBD may be enhanced by coadministration of THC (or vice versa), especially at low (subthreshold) doses [24].

G-Protein-Coupled Receptors (GPCRs): CBD acts at multiple GPCRs, including G-protein-coupled receptor 55 (GPR55), an orphan receptor also thought to be a novel cannabinoid receptor. GPR55 is found in the caudate/putamen and the hippocampus, as well as other peripheral tissues. It is thought to be involved in spatial memory and neural plasticity. Its activation increases intracellular calcium and excitatory neurotransmission in hippocampal neurons. CBD acts as an antagonist at this site, which may contribute to its antiepileptic effects.

Serotonin: CBD enhances serotonergic activity through its actions at the serotonin 1A (5-HT_{1A}) receptor. 5-HT_{1A} has been shown in preclinical studies to be responsible for CBD's antianxiety, antipain, and antiemetic/antinausea effects. Clinical evidence of CBD's efficacy for depression and anxiety is limited, but serotonin reuptake inhibitors are used to treat both conditions, so CBD's therapeutic potential for them (if any) could be mediated by this mechanism [15].

Reactive Oxygen Species: CBD (and other cannabinoids) are potent inhibitors of the formation of reactive oxygen species (ROS). This property was discovered in 1998 and was the basis for a patent (1999) related to cannabinoids' potential neuroprotective effects [25]. Interestingly, among CBD's multiple antitumor effects (shown in vitro and in animal models), it may also *generate* ROS in cancer cells, leading to cytotoxicity or apoptosis or autophagy.

Ion Channels: CBD interacts with multiple ion channels, including the transient receptor potential cation channel subfamily member 1 (TrpV1), also referred to as the capsaicin receptor or vanilloid receptor 1, which is a heat and pain ligand-gated ion channel. This effect may be relevant to CBD's antipain and antiepileptic effects.

Neurotransmitters: Preclinical work shows that CBD interacts directly or indirectly with many neurotransmitter systems, in addition to serotonin. It is known to enhance dopamine D2 receptor signaling, to inhibit adenosine reuptake and act as an agonist at the A1 and A2a receptors, to inhibit glutamate neurotransmission, and to enhance GABA and glycine activity, among others.

Peroxisome Proliferator-Activated Receptors (PPARs): Several studies have documented CBD's role as a PPAR-gamma agonist. PPARs are nuclear hormone receptors that bind to certain segments of DNA to promote or prevent gene transcription. Many of the genes regulated by PPARs are involved in energy metabolism, cell differentiation, and inflammation. CBD may also exert some of its antioxidant properties through this receptor.

In summary, CBD has more than 75 ascribed mechanisms of action (see reviews cited above). While some may be more closely linked to specific therapeutic actions, it may also be the case that combinations and interactions among these various mechanisms contribute to CBD's overall effects.

Unknowns and Concerns: Efficacy, Safety, and Quality

There are now a vast array of products containing CBD that are readily available in the retail and online marketplace. And while CBD appears to be a relatively safe compound, the current environment has created a number of inherent challenges and risks that are borne by the consumer.

Product Quality and Labeling: Although the Farm Bill gave the FDA regulatory authority over CBD products made from cannabis containing less than 0.3% delta-9 THC (i.e., hemp), the sheer number of products and lack of critical safety information have slowed these efforts. The FDA has been seeking information to answer some of the more critical questions related to safety of chronic use in diverse populations, effects on male reproductive function, liver toxicity, driving impairment, alcohol interactions, and dermal penetration. See: https://www.fda.gov/news-events/public-health-focus/information-cbd-data-collection-and-submission.

To address questions related to labeling and associated quality of CBD products, several research groups and the FDA have analyzed the contents of products purported to contain CBD. While the results have varied, they generally show that a majority of products do not contain the amounts of CBD listed on the label, and/or they also contain THC as well as other cannabinoid and noncannabinoid (e.g., lead, arsenic) constituents [26–28].

Furthermore, the FDA has issued warning letters to companies selling CBD products that claim to prevent, diagnose, treat, or cure serious diseases, such as cancer. Some of these products were in further violation of the Federal Food, Drug and Cosmetic (FD&C) Act because they were marketed as dietary supplements, foods, or beverages, which is not permitted as CBD is also an approved medication (Epidiolex®). The FDA also enforces standards of production and manufacturing of products for human consumption, known as current good manufacturing practices (CGMPs), which ensure safety and consistency of products being sold. Without FDA regulation of commercial CBD products, the consumer has no assurances that CGMP practices are being followed.

Dearth of Data: There is much we do not know about the pharmacokinetics, bioavailability, and dosage needs of CBD for different conditions or symptoms. The route of administration is an important consideration, especially related to bioavailability and pharmacokinetics. Dosages that have been used in animal or clinical research can range from 1 to 200 mg/kg/day. Merchandise being sold as wellness products (to promote sleep, counter mild anxiety, or depression, etc.) often contains much lower doses, which may be insufficient to produce purported effects.

As with other substances, CBD's bioavailability or absorption varies with the route of administration. Maximum bioavailability occurs with intravenous administration (100%); followed by inhalation (smoking or vaporization); oral ingestion; and transdermal administration. The onset and duration of effect are also dependent on the route of administration. Currently, the most common route is oral (e.g., Epidiolex®, tinctures) which is subject to first-pass metabolism in the liver. Estimates for Epidiolex® absorption suggest somewhere between 6% and 15% bioavailability. Multiple dosing has been shown to increase absorption, and there are large differences depending on whether the person is fed or fasted, and what they have consumed. High-fat foods can increase CBD absorption up to 5×. Transdermal products are popular, including for treating skin conditions, but there are few data on their depth of penetration. Because CBD is lipophilic, it accumulates in outer layers of the skin and may not penetrate below that. Animal studies indicate that transdermal CBD combined with an enhanced permeator could produce long-lasting behavioral effects in various models of addictive behavior [29].

CBD is metabolized by cytochrome P-450 enzymes, predominantly CYP3A4 and CYP2C19. As a result, it can interfere with the metabolism of other medications using the same enzymatic pathways, potentially resulting in higher-than-recommended blood levels of the affected medications. One example is clobazam, an anticonvulsant used in childhood epilepsy, that may have led to some of the adverse effects associated with Epidiolex® treatment in clinical trials (e.g., increased somnolence), although it does not appear to have contributed to the therapeutic effects. In addition, data from recent studies suggest that CBD modulates SSRI response, including es/citalopram and sertraline [30]. These enzymes are involved in the metabolism of many commonly used medications (and THC) and could result in drug interactions that present risks to certain patient populations. Note that these interactions have only been shown to occur at high CBD doses—typically over 500 mg/day [31].

As noted above, the dosage requirements for different therapeutic indications are largely unknown, and plasma levels are rarely measured in clinical studies. While little toxicity has been reported from even high-dose CBD exposure (up to several grams/day), most studies do not follow participants long enough to determine whether chronic exposure produces additional toxicity. As an FDA-approved medication, Epidiolex® is subject to continued safety monitoring. It is important to note an inverse-U-shaped dose-response curve has been reported for some indications (e.g., anxiety), such that there may be an optimal therapeutic dose range, with effects dropping off (or even reversing) at higher doses.

Notably, the few studies that have looked at repeated CBD administration do not report tolerance development (i.e., the need for higher doses to achieve a therapeutic effect over time), which could be a benefit for clinical treatment. Moreover, CBD does not appear to be converted to THC in humans—also a benefit. And while some CBD users report testing positive for THC on drug screens, that is most likely related to THC contamination of the products they are using, not a metabolic effect.

Despite the wide availability and use of CBD products there are many critical gaps in our knowledge about its safety and efficacy. In addition to those mentioned above, we are lacking data on the impact of long-term use of different products, alone and in combination with other dietary supplements or medications. We are also lacking data on the impact of CBD during critical developmental windows, including fetal development and adolescence. Some research suggests sex-dependent effects, but again very little work has been done in this area. And because this product is developing a large consumer base among adults and older adults, these populations also need to be carefully studied. Towards this end, the FDA is encouraging observational/natural experiments and the use of real-world data/real-world evidence to help provide some answers to guide their regulatory efforts.

Clinical Applications

While CBD is being proposed as a therapeutic intervention for a wide array of conditions, including cancer, autoimmune diseases, nausea and vomiting, and skin diseases, this chapter will focus on its promise for treating neurological and psychiatric disorders, including addiction [32]. As noted earlier, with few exceptions, most of the above-mentioned indications do not have sufficient (or, in some cases, any) clinical data to support their use or FDA approval. Thus, these applications while plausible, and even promising, require further study; some of this research is ongoing (see clinicaltrials.gov).

Notably, CBD does not show abuse liability in preclinical or clinical research, which increases its desirability as a therapeutic option. Preclinical research indicates: no effect on dopamine release (often an indicator of rewarding effects of drugs), no effect on intracranial self-stimulation (ICSS) thresholds (a measure of reward sensitivity), no conditioned place preference (CPP), and no THC drug discriminative effects. In humans, CBD also does not show abuse potential in subjective tests (e.g., drug-liking, feeling high), which led to Epidiolex® originally being placed in Schedule V under the Controlled Substances Act (indicating a low potential for abuse), before being descheduled by the DEA in 2020.

Epilepsy: The FDA approved Epidiolex® in June 2018, which is a cannabis plant extract containing more than 99% CBD in an oral formulation. It has been approved to treat seizures associated with Dravet syndrome, Lennox-Gastaut syndrome, and tuberous sclerosis in patients as young as 1 year old. In most cases, Epidiolex® was added to other treatments that patients were already taking but that failed to adequately control their seizure disorder. More than 1000 patients have participated in placebo-controlled studies for these 3 conditions, in accordance with FDA requirements. Side effects were mostly gastrointestinal (loss of appetite, diarrhea, nausea, vomiting), but elevation of liver enzymes (suggesting potential liver damage), headaches, and increased sleepiness were also reported. These risks were considered acceptable relative to the severity of the illnesses being treated. These patients continue to be monitored for potential long-term effects of exposure. Doses used vary and are titrated for optimal therapeutic effect. They can be as high as 25 mg/kg/day, but starting doses are in the range of 5 mg/kg/day [33]. Other research is ongoing to determine whether Epidiolex® (or other pharmaceutical formulations of CBD) would be useful for other types of seizure disorders.

Pain: Although pain is the most commonly reported reason for medical use of cannabis products, most of the clinical research has been conducted with THC (marinol or dronabinol) or THC-predominant plant products. The sole exception is nabiximols (Sativex), a plant-derived oromucosal spray, containing 2.7 mg THC and 2.5 mg CBD per spray. Sativex is an approved medication in several European Countries and Canada, but not in the U.S. It is approved for treating neuropathic pain and spasticity associated with multiple sclerosis, and (in some countries) cancer pain that is unresponsive to opioids.

CBD has potent anti-inflammatory properties, which could produce relief from certain types of pain, especially in conditions characterized by chronic neuropathic pain and inflammation (e.g., irritable bowel syndrome and arthritis). To date most of the clinical research does *not* support a role for CBD on its own for acute or chronic pain conditions, with the exception of certain types of facial pain for which topical application can be used. Also, preclinical research suggests CBD might potentiate THC's or morphine's antinociceptive effects, and its contribution to the antipain effects of Sativex remains to be determined.

Anxiety: CBD's potential to alleviate anxiety has received a lot of attention and anecdotal support, although there are few studies in clinical populations. In several preclinical research paradigms, CBD has consistently been shown to have effects similar to other antianxiety medications (benzodiazepines, antidepressants), and these appear related to its $5HT_{1A}$ agonist properties [15]. In some rodent studies, effects were seen only in "pre-stressed" animals, suggesting that CBD might be more effective in subjects with higher-than-normal baseline levels of stress.

A number of studies have evaluated CBD's antianxiety effects in healthy controls subjected to an anxiety-provoking situation [7]. The situation most often used, and with the most consistent beneficial effects for CBD, is a simulated public speaking task. CBD's effects were, in some instances, dose-dependent, with moderate doses (e.g., 300 mg, oral capsule) being more effective than low or high doses (100 mg, and 600 or 900 mg, respectively), although doses used in clinical populations to achieve an antianxiety effect were higher. Data from these studies suggest that CBD was not effective in all anxiety paradigms; thus there may be certain conditions or degrees of stress necessary for its effect to manifest. Clinical studies are ongoing in patients with various anxiety disorders.

Studies also suggest CBD may be useful for patients with posttraumatic stress disorder (PTSD). PTSD involves a powerful learned response, such that environmental stimuli associated with a prior trauma evoke severe distress long after they no longer predict negative outcomes. Conditioned fear in animals, involving repeated pairing of a neutral stimulus (e.g., a light) with an aversive one (e.g., foot shock), is a model of the type of learning that contributes to the development of PTSD. This type of learning can be resistant to extinction training, which decouples the environmental stimulus and the traumatic event, although that is the basis of exposure therapy. Drugs that can interfere with or blunt the learning of the response or facilitate its extinction (e.g., attenuate an animal's freezing behavior after the light is no longer predictive of foot shock) may be useful in treating PTSD. CBD has been shown to do this in various preclinical paradigms. There are also a few studies in humans that support the idea that CBD can facilitate extinction learning and can affect the brain circuits thought to be involved in responses to anxiety. There are also case reports supporting the use of CBD in PTSD, but again clinical trials are needed [34]. CBD may also be helpful for sleep, which is frequently disrupted in patients with PTSD, although the data supporting this are minimal. CBD's effects may be dose dependent, with lower doses being stimulatory and higher doses, sedating.

Thus, with further research to clarify its effects, CBD may represent an adjunctive treatment for PTSD and its symptoms [35].

Psychotic Disorders: Psychotic disorders, including schizophrenia, are among the most disabling mental health disorders, usually beginning in late adolescence or early adulthood. As noted above, CBD is thought to counter the psychotogenic effects of THC and might have a role in treating psychotic disorders. Animal models of psychosis are limited, in part because of the nature of the symptoms and the complexity of the disease as well as an incomplete understanding of its etiology. There are several neurodevelopmental models (e.g., maternal immune activation during gestation; late gestational administration of the antimitotic agent, methylazoxymethanol acetate (MAM); and the spontaneously hypertensive rat strain), all of which produce a phenotype in mice or rats during adulthood that model some aspects of schizophrenia. In adolescent or adult animals, a commonly used model involves MK-801 disruption of prepulse inhibition (PPI). MK-801 is an NMDA glutamate antagonist, which produces hyperactivity, stereotypy (repetitive non-goal-directed movements), and a deficit in PPI. PPI involves the presentation of 2 sounds in close succession: an initial weak stimulus (prepulse) followed by a stronger one that causes an acute startle response. Under normal conditions, the prepulse dampens the response to the subsequent stronger one. Disruption of PPI is thought to model stimulus gating deficits (failure to ignore irrelevant stimuli) reported in people with schizophrenia. CBD can reverse this effect, as well as the hyperlocomotion and stereotypy produced by NMDA antagonists and dopamine agonists.

Another interesting approach relates to the use of CBD as a prevention or early intervention strategy for psychotic disorders in those at high risk or showing subthreshold symptoms. There are data suggesting that such an approach could be beneficial; however, care must be exercised in the type of preventative treatment used, since a majority of those with prodromal symptoms or at high risk will not go on to develop schizophrenia. In that regard, CBD as a mostly nontoxic substance, if effective, would have significant advantages over current antipsychotic medications. While this has not yet been tested in humans, the use of neurodevelopmental animal models such as those described above has presented an opportunity to test this hypothesis and has shown positive results with prolonged administration of CBD at relatively high doses (e.g., 30–60 mg/kg/day) [36].

Clinical studies using CBD in patients with schizophrenia have produced inconsistent results. In many studies, CBD is used as an add-on to other antipsychotic medications, with relative safety even at high doses (more than 1G/day); in several clinical trials, CBD was beneficial in reducing the positive symptoms (hallucinations, delusions, disorganized thinking) but less effective on the cognitive or negative symptoms (e.g., social withdrawal). This remains a promising area of research, and there are multiple clinical trials attempting to demonstrate CBD's potential as an antipsychotic medication.

Addiction: There are multiple preclinical models for various aspects of addiction. Self-administration involves the voluntary intake of substances. Variations of this paradigm measure the motivation an animal has to acquire the drug or whether they will develop a "compulsive" pattern of intake. For some drugs, characteristic withdrawal behaviors can be modeled. Other models rely on classical conditioning by pairing a stimulus or an environment with the drug or the prediction of the drug's availability and measuring the animal's preference for that stimulus/environment. Finally, there are models of "relapse" based on known triggers of relapse in people with substance use disorders, such as exposure to a small amount of a drug (priming), cues that are associated with the drug or that predict its availability, and stress exposure. These models have been used to test CBD's potential to treat substance use disorders.

In general, CBD does not prevent self-administration of most substances (with the possible exception of alcohol and stimulants at high CBD doses). Rather its effects seem to be more prominent in cue and stress-induced relapse models, for opioids, alcohol, and cocaine. In a rodent study by Gonzalez-Cuevas et al. (2019), a transdermal preparation of CBD administered for 7 days at 24-hour intervals reduced context- and stress-induced drug reinstatement for cocaine and alcohol, and this effect lasted for up to 5 months [37]. Plasma and brain levels of CBD were not detectable after 3 days. In this study, other behaviors often associated with relapse (e.g., general anxiety and impulsivity) were also measured and similarly dampened by CBD. An earlier study showed similar effects of CBD on cue-induced heroin seeking (10 and 20 mg/kg. i.p.), but not priming or extinction of heroin self-administration. This effect was observed at 24 h and 2 weeks after CBD administration and was associated with the normalization of several brain markers of cue-induced heroin self-administration in the mesolimbic nervous system.

These promising preclinical studies led Hurd et al. to conduct a randomized double-blind placebo-controlled trial in abstinent heroin users ($N = 42$ males and females) evaluating CBD's effect on cue-induced craving and anxiety. CBD [Epidiolex® (400 or 800 mg)] or placebo was administered once daily for 3 days, and participants were tested 1 h after their last dose and then 24 h and 1 week later. Both cue-induced craving and anxiety were reduced by CBD treatment, as well as physiological indicators of anxiety (heart rate and cortisol levels) [38, 39]. There was no difference by dose of CBD, and there were few adverse effects. Follow-up studies are planned or in progress to determine whether CBD could be an effective treatment for opioid use disorders.

With respect to other substances, preclinical research suggests potential benefits of CBD for preventing alcohol-withdrawal-induced seizures (in mice) and for protecting against neurotoxicity and liver damage using binge models of alcohol intake. And some clinical research supports effectiveness of nabiximols for cannabis withdrawal symptoms but not for promoting abstinence; the role of CBD in these effects has not been determined. Recently, a small clinical study by Freemen et al. (2020) suggested that CBD (400 mg and 800 mg) was safe and more efficacious than placebo at reducing cannabis use [40]. Case report data also suggest a role for CBD in tobacco cessation. CBD's antianxiety effects may contribute to many of the observed beneficial effects, particularly in patients experiencing substance withdrawal.

Conclusions

CBD is a remarkably versatile compound with more than 75 putative mechanisms of action and an equally wide array of potential therapeutic uses, including in illnesses for which there are no or few alternatives. Its safety profile is quite good over a range of doses, it is not intoxicating or addictive, and for these and other reasons it has become extremely popular with the public with an equally active and successful supplier industry.

Currently, there is only one FDA-approved CBD medication (Epidiolex®) that is used to treat severe seizure disorders in children. Nevertheless, CBD is being added to foods and beverages and is available in dietary supplements, tinctures, cosmetics, transdermal preparations, and many more products implicitly or explicitly promising improved health or wellness. In general, the doses in these products are lower than those tested in clinical trials. These products are unregulated, and most are illegal under the FD&C Act, which does not allow medications to be added to food or beverages or to be sold as dietary supplements. The FDA could consider an exemption for CBD products, once it has accrued sufficient safety data. FDA regulation could help ensure that CBD is manufactured using CGMPs, and with appropriate product labeling.

At this time, most of the data supporting CBD's therapeutic potential comes from preclinical science—both in vitro and in vivo—and there are very few completed clinical trials. The dosages required for treatment of various conditions are unknown, vary widely, and in some cases may fall within a narrow therapeutic window. Bioavailability varies by route of administration and whether the individual is fed or fasted. A number of studies suggest long-lasting effects of CBD beyond the window of its bioavailability, which could indicate a triggering of epigenetic or other molecular changes that sustain its effects. Most studies do not report tolerance to CBD's therapeutic effects, but few have been carried out long enough to determine whether this is the case. Sex and age effects are unknown, including effects during vulnerable periods such as prenatal development. There are known risks, including CBD's interactions with other drugs or medications due to its metabolism by cytochrome P-450 enzymes. In clinical studies with Epidiolex®, patients also report GI symptoms, headaches, and possible effects on the liver.

While CBD may counter some of THC's more serious adverse effects (e.g., psychosis, cognitive impairment), a direct relationship has been difficult to demonstrate in human laboratory studies and may depend on dosing, route of administration, timing, and source (e.g., whether CBD is a component of a plant product being used and what the ratio of THC to CBD is). CBD may also potentiate THC's beneficial effects, for instance in alleviating pain, in preventing and treating chemotherapy-induced nausea, and in cell culture and/or animal studies of several types of cancer.

The complicated and evolving legal and regulatory framework has presented barriers for conducting research with CBD, including clinical trials; and there is an urgent need for safety and efficacy data for the wide variety of conditions CBD is alleged to treat. Caution should be exercised in the use of currently marketed products since adequate oversight is lacking and, in many cases, there are insufficient data on dosing and safety. Physicians should be prudent in making recommendations to their patients and ensure that they are aware of the risks associated with purchasing unregulated products and of using these products in lieu of known effective treatments for their conditions when such treatments are available.

Highlights Box 3.1 Key Points in Patient Psychoeducation

- CBD is a non-intoxicating component of the cannabis plant that may have therapeutic uses in multiple psychiatric and neurological disorders.
- Epidiolex® is the only FDA-approved CBD medication. It is used for the treatment of severe seizure disorders.
- CBD's overall safety profile is quite good, although questions remain regarding long-term use; use by certain populations (e.g., pregnant women); and drug interactions due to its metabolism by cytochrome P-450 enzymes.
- Most data supporting CBD's myriad therapeutic effects are preclinical—both in vitro and in vivo—with few large clinical trials. Many are underway: see clinicaltrials.gov.
- A wide variety of unregulated CBD products are available in the consumer market. These products do not have FDA oversight; some are inaccurately labeled (e.g., containing THC), or may be manufactured under conditions that do not meet good manufacturing practice (GMP) standards.
- Physicians should be prudent in making recommendations to patients; consumers should educate themselves on the risks of using unregulated products, especially in lieu of known effective treatments.

CBD type	Description
Epidiolex® (plant-derived CBD)	• Not scheduled • FDA-approved treatment for severe seizure disorders: Lennox-Gastaut syndrome, Dravet syndrome, tuberous sclerosis complex, in patients 1 year or older • Plant derived (marijuana) • Oral solution
Hemp-sourced CBD	• Not scheduled • Defined as cannabis sativa plant with <0.3% delta-9 THC (dry weight) • Subject to FDA regulation[a] – Hemp seed and hemp seed oil (which contain neither THC nor CBD) can be sold as food products – Hemp derived CBD cannot be added to food products, or sold as a dietary supplement, since CBD is the main active component of a medication – Labeling and marketing requirements[a] – Good manufacturing process (GMP) production[a] • Widely available through common sources, with no FDA oversight of products • Available in multiple forms: Tinctures, edibles, gels, capsules, vaping liquids, transdermal preparations, suppositories, etc.
Dispensary products	• Schedule I, unless hemp derived • Source may be hemp or marijuana • Intended use may be medical or nonmedical • May contain varying amounts of THC • Regulations vary by state • Available in multiple forms (as above)
Synthetic CBD	• Schedule I • Not yet available: Under development as medication

[a]FDA has not yet exerted its full regulatory authority over most CBD products.

Strength of the evidence for CBD or combined CBD/THC (i.e., Sativex) neurological/psychological indications	
Indication	Strength of evidence
Epilepsy (Epidiolex®)	High
Pain (cancer pain; pain associated with multiple sclerosis) (Sativex®: Oromucosal spray containing 2.5 mg CBD/2.7 mg THC/100 μl dose)	High[a]
Anxiety	Moderate
Psychosis/psychotic disorders	Moderate/mixed
Addiction (alcohol, tobacco, cannabis, opioids)	Low

[a]Sativex is approved in multiple countries, but not in the U.S., for these indications. CBD role in therapeutic effect is undetermined.

References

1. Adams R, Hunt M, Clark JH. Structure of cannabidiol, a product isolated from the marihuana extract of Minnesota wild hemp. J Am Chem Soc. 1940;62(1):196–200.
2. Mechoulam R, Shvo Y. Hashish. I. The structure of cannabidiol. Tetrahedron. 1963;19(12):2073–8.
3. Carlini EA, Leite JR, Tannhauser M, Berardi AC. Cannabidiol and Cannabis sativa extract protect mice and rats against convulsive agents. J Pharm Pharmacol. 1973;25(8):664–5.
4. Izquierdo I, Orsingher OA, Berardi AC. Effect of cannabidiol and of other Cannabis sativa compounds on hippocampal seizure discharges. Psychopharmacologia. 1973;28(1):95–102.
5. Cunha JM, Carlini EA, Pereira AE, Ramos OL, Pimentel C, Gagliardi R, et al. Chronic Administration of Cannabidiol to healthy volunteers and epileptic patients. Pharmacology. 1980;21(3):175–85.
6. Weed: Dr. Sanjay Gupta Reports premieres Sunday, 8/11 8p ET [Internet]. [cited 2021 Apr 24]. https://cnnpressroom.blogs.cnn.com/2013/08/05/weed-drsanjaygupta-reports-premieres-on-cnn-sunday-august-11-at-8-pm-et/
7. Crippa JA, Zuardi AW, Martín-Santos R, Bhattacharyya S, Atakan Z, McGuire P, et al. Cannabis and anxiety: a critical review of the evidence. Hum Psychopharmacol Clin Exp. 2009;24(7):515–23.
8. Conaway KM. H.R.2 - 115th Congress (2017–2018): Agriculture Improvement Act of 2018 [Internet]. 2018 [cited 2021 Apr 22]. https://www.congress.gov/bill/115th-congress/house-bill/2
9. Office of the Federal Register, National Archives and Records Administration. (2020, August 20). 85 FR 51639 - Implementation of the Agriculture Improvement Act of 2018. [Government]. Office of the Federal Register, National Archives and Records Administration https://www.govinfo.gov/app/details/FR-2020-08-21/2020-17356
10. Food & Drug Administration. (2021, Jan 22). FDA Regulation of Cannabis and Cannabis-Derived Products, Including Cannabidiol (CBD). FDA [Internet]. [cited 2021 Apr 22]. https://www.fda.gov/news-events/public-health-focus/fda-regulation-cannabis-and-cannabis-derived-products-including-cannabidiol-cbd
11. Legislative news, studies and analysis | National Conference of State Legislatures [Internet]. [cited 2021 Apr 22]. https://www.ncsl.org/
12. de Almeida DL, Devi LA. Diversity of molecular targets and signaling pathways for CBD. Pharmacol Res Perspect. 2020;8(6):e00682.
13. Devinsky O, Cilio MR, Cross H, Fernandez-Ruiz J, French J, Hill C, et al. Cannabidiol: pharmacology and potential therapeutic role in epilepsy and other neuropsychiatric disorders. Epilepsia. 2014 Jun;55(6):791–802.
14. Scarante FF, Ribeiro MA, Almeida-Santos AF, Guimarães FS, Campos AC. Glial cells and their contribution to the mechanisms of action of Cannabidiol in neuropsychiatric disorders. Front Pharmacol. 2021;11:618065. https://www.ncbi.nlm.nih.gov/pmc/articles/PMC7890128/
15. Melas PA, Scherma M, Fratta W, Cifani C, Fadda P. Cannabidiol as a potential treatment for anxiety and mood disorders: molecular targets and epigenetic insights from preclinical research. Int J Mol Sci. 2021;22(4):1863.
16. Elmes MW, Kaczocha M, Berger WT, Leung K, Ralph BP, Wang L, et al. Fatty acid-binding proteins (FABPs) are intracellular carriers for Δ9-tetrahydrocannabinol (THC) and cannabidiol (CBD). J Biol Chem. 2015;290(14):8711–21.
17. Criscuolo E, De Sciscio ML, Fezza F, Maccarrone M. In silico and in vitro analysis of major cannabis-derived compounds as fatty acid amide hydrolase inhibitors. Molecules. 2020;26(1):48. https://www.ncbi.nlm.nih.gov/pmc/articles/PMC7795171/
18. Morgan CJA, Curran HV. Effects of cannabidiol on schizophrenia-like symptoms in people who use cannabis. Br J Psychiatry. 2008;192(4):306–7.
19. Di Forti M, Quattrone D, Freeman TP, Tripoli G, Gayer-Anderson C, Quigley H, et al. The contribution of cannabis use to variation in the incidence of psychotic disorder across Europe (EU-GEI): a multicentre case-control study. Lancet Psychiatry. 2019;6(5):427–36.

20. Morgan CJA, Schafer G, Freeman TP, Curran HV. Impact of cannabidiol on the acute memory and psychotomimetic effects of smoked cannabis: naturalistic study: naturalistic study [corrected]. Br J Psychiatry J Ment Sci. 2010;197(4):285–90.
21. Morgan CJ, Freeman TP, Schafer GL, Curran HV. Cannabidiol attenuates the appetitive effects of Δ9-tetrahydrocannabinol in humans smoking their chosen cannabis. Neuropsychopharmacology. 2010;35(9):1879–85.
22. Freeman AM, Petrilli K, Lees R, Hindocha C, Mokrysz C, Curran HV, et al. How does cannabidiol (CBD) influence the acute effects of delta-9-tetrahydrocannabinol (THC) in humans? A systematic review. Neurosci Biobehav Rev. 2019;107:696–712.
23. Englund A, Freeman TP, Murray RM, McGuire P. Can we make cannabis safer? Lancet Psychiatry. 2017;4(8):643–8.
24. Nutt DJ, Phillips LD, Barnes MP, Brander B, Curran HV, Fayaz A, et al. A multicriteria decision analysis comparing pharmacotherapy for chronic neuropathic pain, including cannabinoids and cannabis-based medical products. Cannabis Cannabinoid Res. 2021; Mar 17 [cited 2021 Aug 19]. https://www.liebertpub.com/doi/full/10.1089/can.2020.0129
25. Hampson AJ, Grimaldi M, Axelrod J, Wink D. Cannabidiol and (−)Δ9-tetrahydrocannabinol are neuroprotective antioxidants. Proc Natl Acad Sci. 1998;95(14):8268–73.
26. Bonn-Miller MO, Loflin MJE, Thomas BF, Marcu JP, Hyke T, Vandrey R. Labeling accuracy of Cannabidiol extracts sold online. JAMA. 2017;318(17):1708–9.
27. Hazekamp A. The trouble with CBD oil. Med Cannabis Cannabinoids. 2018;1(1):65–72.
28. Liebling JP, Clarkson NJ, Gibbs BW, Yates AS, O'Sullivan SE. An analysis of over-the-counter Cannabidiol products in the United Kingdom. Cannabis Cannabinoid Res. 2020 Apr 1 [cited 2021 Apr 22]. https://www.liebertpub.com/doi/full/10.1089/can.2019.0078
29. Prud'homme M, Cata R, Jutras-Aswad D. Cannabidiol as an intervention for addictive behaviors: a systematic review of the evidence. Subst Abuse. 2015;9:33–8.
30. Anderson LL, Doohan PT, Oldfield L, Kevin RC, Arnold JC, Berger M, et al. Citalopram and Cannabidiol: in vitro and in vivo evidence of pharmacokinetic interactions relevant to the treatment of anxiety disorders in young people. J Clin Psychopharmacol. 41(5):525–33. https://journals.lww.com/psychopharmacology/Abstract/9000/Citalopram_and_Cannabidiol__In_Vitro_and_In_Vivo.98295.aspx
31. Brown JD, Winterstein AG. Potential adverse drug events and drug–drug interactions with medical and consumer cannabidiol (CBD) use. J Clin Med. 2019;8(7):989.
32. Mechoulam R, Parker LA, Gallily R. Cannabidiol: an overview of some pharmacological aspects. J Clin Pharmacol. 2002;42(S1):11S–9S.
33. Trial of cannabidiol for drug-resistant seizures in the Dravet syndrome | NEJM [Internet]. [cited 2021 Apr 22]. https://www.nejm.org/doi/full/10.1056/nejmoa1611618
34. Elms L, Shannon S, Hughes S, Lewis N. Cannabidiol in the treatment of post-traumatic stress disorder: a case series. J Altern Complement Med. 2019;25(4):392–7.
35. Bitencourt RM, Pamplona FA, Takahashi RN. Facilitation of contextual fear memory extinction and anti-anxiogenic effects of AM404 and cannabidiol in conditioned rats. Eur Neuropsychopharmacol. 2008;18(12):849–59.
36. Loss CM, Teodoro L, Rodrigues GD, Moreira LR, Peres FF, Zuardi AW, et al. Is Cannabidiol during neurodevelopment a promising therapy for schizophrenia and autism Spectrum disorders? Front Pharmacol. 2021;11:635763. https://www.ncbi.nlm.nih.gov/pmc/articles/PMC7890086/
37. Unique treatment potential of cannabidiol for the prevention of relapse to drug use: preclinical proof of principle | Neuropsychopharmacology [Internet]. [cited 2021 Apr 22]. https://www.nature.com/articles/s41386-018-0050-8
38. Hurd YL, Spriggs S, Alishayev J, Winkel G, Gurgov K, Kudrich C, et al. Cannabidiol for the reduction of cue-induced craving and anxiety in drug-abstinent individuals with heroin use disorder: a double-blind randomized placebo-controlled trial. Am J Psychiatry. 2019;176(11):911–22.

39. Early phase in the development of cannabidiol as a treatment for addiction: opioid relapse takes initial center stage | SpringerLink [Internet]. [cited 2021 Apr 22]. https://link.springer.com/article/10.1007/s13311-015-0373-7
40. Freeman TP, Hindocha C, Baio G, Shaban NDC, Thomas EM, Astbury D, et al. Cannabidiol for the treatment of cannabis use disorder: a phase 2a, double-blind, placebo-controlled, randomised, adaptive Bayesian trial. Lancet Psychiatry. 2020;7(10):865–74.

Part II

Cannabis in Child and Adolescent Mental Health Settings

Developmental Impact

4

Jesse D. Hinckley and John Dillon

Introduction

The endocannabinoid system (ECS) is the primary endogenous system through which exogenous cannabinoids act. Please see Chap. 1 for a review of the outlines the components of the endocannabinoid system. The ECS is a highly evolutionarily conserved system, which suggests the developmental processes modulated by the ECS are vital for normal development. As reviewed by Harkany et al., the ECS is present from the earliest stages of pregnancy and regulates key aspects of fertilization and implantation [1]. Anandamide (AEA), a primary endocannabinoid, facilitates fertilization through cannabis 1 receptors (CB1R) expressed on spermatozoa. Subsequently, transient reductions in AEA in the uterus and CB1R and CB2R expression in the embryo facilitate blastocyst activation and enable implantation into the uterine wall.

Neurodevelopment

As the fetus continues to develop, the ECS also plays a fundamental role in regulating multiple stages of brain development (neurodevelopment) and modulates the mature nervous system throughout adulthood (Highlights Box 4.1) [1–3]. Neurodevelopment begins early in embryogenesis and continues through young adulthood, presenting a uniquely vulnerable time to the detrimental effects of cannabis use (Fig. 4.1). Throughout neurodevelopment, CB1R is widely expressed and is one of the most abundant G-protein-coupled receptors in the brain [1, 3]. CB1R is detectable in the human fetal brain at approximately 14 weeks gestation. Expression progressively increases in a temporally and spatially regulated pattern in the cerebral cortex, caudate nucleus, putamen, cerebellar cortex, hippocampus,

J. D. Hinckley (✉) · J. Dillon
Department of Psychiatry, University of Colorado School of Medicine, Aurora, CO, USA
e-mail: jesse.hinckley@cuanschutz.edu; john.dillon@cuanschutz.edu

P. Riggs, T. Thant (eds.), *Cannabis in Psychiatric Practice*, Psychiatry Update 3,
https://doi.org/10.1007/978-3-031-04874-6_4

Highlights Box 4.1 Key Points in Neurodevelopment

- The ECS is an important regulator of fetal development from conception.
- The ECS regulates many aspects of brain development, including organization of the brain into mature neural circuits, which continues until about 25 years old.
- The ECS also mediates development of neurotransmitters important to cognitive function and mental health, including glutamate, serotonin, dopamine, and opioid systems.
- Behavioral functions regulated ECS signaling include cognition, learning and memory, attention, drug/addictive behaviors, social interactions, pain sensitivity, sexual behavior, and stress response.
- Over the lifespan, the ECS continues to mediate behavioral functions and the ability of the brain to learn and adapt, forming new memories and refining learned functions.

and amygdala. Further, endocannabinoids are "made on demand," facilitating maintenance of a precise temporal and spatial pattern of signaling [1, 3]. 2-arachidonoylglycerol (2-AG) concentrations are 1000-fold higher throughout brain development, setting a basal tone for the ECS. Conversely, AEA levels are relatively low at midgestation and gradually increase throughout the perinatal period and into adolescence.

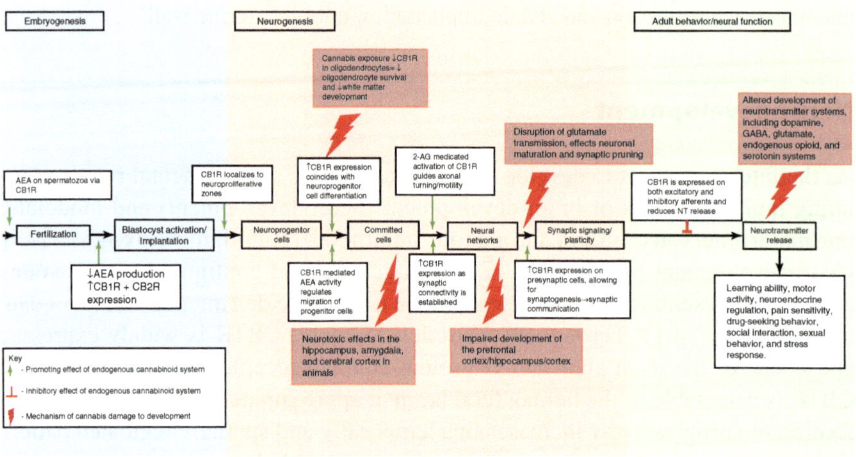

Fig. 4.1 The effects of prenatal cannabis exposure throughout neurodevelopment. Stages of development during embryogenesis, ongoing neurogenesis, and adult neural function are presented. The stages of neurogenesis are presented sequentially for simplicity. It is important to note these stages take place simultaneously and at different times and rates throughout the developing brain. White boxes show the role of and changes in the endocannabinoid system across development. Key points of exogenous cannabis exposure are presented in the red boxes

Neuromaturation: Neurogenesis, Synaptogenesis, and Myelination

Development of the brain begins with a collection of neuronal progenitor cells, which must migrate to specific locations in the brain, differentiate to specific types of neurons (neuronal differentiation), and form a network of connections or synapses. Synaptic pruning then refines connections to establish neuronal circuits. The ECS regulates many aspects of neuronal differentiation, including neurogenesis, neuronal migration, neurite outgrowth, and axonal pathfinding (Fig. 4.1) [1, 4]. Temporal and spatial expression of endocannabinoids and receptors is also important in maintaining homeostatic control of synaptic transmission in the developmental brain in a narrow physiological time window [5].

Endocannabinoid signaling, particularly AEA-mediated signaling, regulates survival of and differentiation of neuronal progenitor cells, ensuring adequate quantities of cells during neurodevelopment [1]. CB1R localizes to cell proliferative regions including the subventricular zones of the striatum, nucleus accumbens, and neocortex [6, 7]. There is a robust upregulation of CB1R expression that coincides with commitment of neuronal progenitor cells to differentiate, and endocannabinoid signaling subsequently mediates acquisition of neuronal identity and initial organization of neural networks [6]. As development continues the distribution of CB1R shifts to the cerebral cortex, coinciding with neuronal cell migration through the cortex to their final target site [2]. Through CB1R signaling, AEA is proposed to regulate migration of progenitor cells and neurons into the cortical plate, as well as long-distance migration of interneurons [4].

As neurons reach their target sites and development progresses, CB1R expression increases on axons and axonal growth cones along developing axonal trajectories, or white matter [1]. CB1R levels subsequently peak when synaptic connectivity is established [7]. CB1 receptors cluster at anchor points in immature neuronal networks to facilitate information processing. As neurons reach their destination, axonal growth cones orchestrate axon tract development. 2-AG-mediated activation of CB1R in axonal growth cones helps guide directional turning and impacts motility of the developing axon [8].

These CB1R expression sites along axons are termed "atypical" because this is a unique distribution pattern that only exists in the developing brain and is essentially absent from the fully developed brain [2]. Considering these unique developmental expression patterns, endocannabinoid-mediated signaling is widely implicated in the organization of long-range axon tract development including corticothalamic and corticospinal tracts [3, 4]. The role of the ECS in axonal guidance is supported by animal studies, which demonstrate deletion or blockade of CB1R results in increased aberrant axon trajectories in the corpus callosum and abnormal fasciculations of long-range axons [3, 4]. As axonal fasciculations and pathways develop, 2-AG mediates activation of radial glial cells and oligodendrocytes to regulate myelination, further establishing mature neural circuits [4].

As neural circuits form, CB1R expression is enriched on presynaptic neurons [1, 3]. Endocannabinoid-mediated retrograde signaling at central synapses allows control of the earliest events of presynaptic neurotransmitter release during the transition from synaptogenesis to synaptic communication in developing neuronal circuits [6]. This pattern of expression continues in the adult brain, enabling ECS-mediated regulation of synaptic transmission and of adult synaptic plasticity [6].

Neurotransmitter System Development

As with neuronal circuit formation, the ECS also mediates development of multiple neurotransmitter systems (Box 4.1). CB1R is expressed on glutamatergic, cholinergic, glycinergic, and serotonergic neurons [4]. ECS signaling also targets other neurotransmitters, including dopamine, orexin A, adenosine 2A, and delta and mu opioid receptors. Interestingly, dopaminergic, or tyrosine hydroxylase (TH)-containing, neurons express CB1R only during neurodevelopment [2]. CB1R is expressed on both excitatory and inhibitory afferents, and endocannabinoid-mediated signaling generally decreases neurotransmitter release [6]. Through these neurotransmitter systems, the ECS mediates several behavioral functions, including learning ability, motor activity, neuroendocrine regulation, and pain sensitivity, as well as drug-seeking behavior, social interaction, sexual behavior, and stress response.

Neurodevelopmental Impact of Cannabinoid Exposure

Determining the neurodevelopmental impact of cannabinoid exposure is complicated by cannabinoid pharmacodynamics, developmental timing of exposure, overall dose and duration of exposure, and gender, among other factors.

Cannabinoid Potency and Timing of Exposure

Whereas endocannabinoid signaling lasts seconds, exposure to exogenous cannabinoids, such as smoking or ingestion of cannabis, results in more sustained (minutes to hours) and much more indiscriminate signaling patterns [4]. Further, the potency of cannabinoids varies dramatically between cannabis products. Tetrahydrocannabinol (THC), the primary psychoactive cannabinoid, is a potent, low-efficacy cannabinoid receptor agonist that outcompetes endocannabinoids for receptor binding [6]. On the other hand, cannabidiol (CBD), a primary cannabinoid of pharmaceutical or medical interest, is a negative allosteric modulator of CB1R and attenuates activation by THC and endocannabinoids. Like THC, synthetic cannabinoids exhibit high potency and high efficacy. The physiologic and neurodevelopmental impacts of varying formulations of cannabinoid concentrations and ratios are not well understood.

Animal models allow more controlled experimental settings, where researchers determine the timing, formulation, dose, and duration of exposure, when compared to human consumption of cannabis. These animal studies provided initial insights that neurodevelopment is a unique period of vulnerability to the detrimental effects of cannabinoids on the brain [9]. As reviewed by Lubman and Schneider, exposure to exogenous cannabinoids during neurodevelopment results in impairments of neuronal differentiation and survival, alterations in neurotransmitter system development, cognitive impairments, hyperactivity, cross-tolerance with other illicit drugs and alterations to the opioid system, and learning and memory deficits (Highlights Box 4.2) [9, 10]. Animals exposed to cannabinoids during neurodevelopment, comparable to childhood through young adulthood, show continued neurocognitive impairments, even after periods of abstinence. However, animals who are exposed to cannabinoids after completion of neurodevelopment, comparable to adulthood after approximately 25 years old, do not exhibit similar vulnerabilities.

Highlights Box 4.2 Cognitive Effects of Cannabis Exposure

- Endocannabinoids are made "on demand" to maintain tight temporal and spatial signaling lasting seconds.
- Exogenous cannabinoid exposure results in sustained, indiscriminate signaling.
- Cannabis exposure during neurodevelopment impairs neural circuit formation and neuron survival and alters development of neurotransmitter systems.
- Affected behavioral functions include cognition, learning and memory, emotional reactivity, drug-seeking/addictive behavior, and depression and anxiety.

Prenatal exposure

- Teratogenicity: fetal growth restriction and lower birth weight for gestational age.
- Infancy: increased startle response and irritability, altered sleep patterns.
- Childhood: short-term memory and verbal reasoning impairment, deficits in sustained attention, and increased hyperactivity and impulsivity, as well as higher rates of depression.
- Adolescents: changes in attentional behavior and adaptive learning and higher rates of depression and problematic substance use.

Adolescent exposure

- Brain development continues through young adulthood (about age 25 years old).
- Imaging studies show changes in brain structure and connectivity.
- Impacts psychomotor speed (athletics and driving), complex attention, learning and memory, abstract reasoning, decision making, processing speed, attention, and working memory.

- Associated with higher rates of depression, anxiety, and psychosis.
- Cannabis use at least 4 days per week is associated with decrease in full-scale IQ of approximately 8 points, lower grade point average, and poorer scholastic aptitude test scores.
- Cannabis use of 10 days a month is associated with increased risky and impulsive decision making.
- Earlier age of onset, duration of use, and frequency of use increase risk of negative cognitive impacts.
- Impairments in executive functioning persist even in abstinence.

Mechanisms of Exogenous Cannabinoid Exposure

The increased vulnerability to the detrimental effects of cannabinoids during fetal development is likely due to the vital roles of the ECS in modulating neurodevelopment. One mechanism of exogenous cannabinoid exposure is downregulation of CB1R, which is observed to a much higher degree in the developing brain [11]. Prolonged cannabis exposure downregulates CB1R in oligodendrocytes, which may impact oligodendrocyte survival, resulting in decreased myelination and altered white matter development. Additionally, prenatal cannabinoid exposure disrupts glutamate transmission, which regulates neuronal maturation and synaptic pruning [9]. Cannabinoid exposure also alters expression of genes that regulate neuron proliferation, migration, and synaptogenesis [12].

Exogenous cannabinoid exposure also impacts the development of neurotransmitter systems, including dopamine, GABA, glutamate, endogenous opioid, and serotonin systems [2, 4]. To better understand how cannabis exposure during pregnancy impacts the development of neurotransmitter systems, the Hurd lab characterized midgestational fetal brains [7, 13]. Maternal cannabis use is associated with a reduction of dopamine D2 receptor density in the amygdala in a dose-dependent manner, such that moderate to high cannabis use ($\geq$0.4 joints/day) is associated with the lowest levels of D2 receptor expression [7]. The frontostriatopallidal proenkephalin/D2 receptor circuit maps onto inhibitory control behavior, and downregulation predicts more impulsive behavior in cannabis-exposed offspring. Changes in enkephalin/D2 receptor density in the amygdala and nucleus accumbens, which mediate emotion and reward, are also implicated in depression, drug addiction, and schizophrenia [14]. Reward and addictive behaviors are also modulated by interactions between the ECS and opioid system [7]. Particularly proenkephalin containing neurons, which target mu and delta opioid receptors, are sensitive to prenatal THC exposure. Animal studies also support this predisposition for substance use, with offspring exposed to cannabis in utero demonstrating increased impulsivity and self-administration of heroin and cocaine, which is associated with alterations in metabolic activity in the frontal lobe and amygdala [7].

Teratogenicity of Exogenous Cannabinoids

In addition to the central nervous system, the ECS is expressed as a regulatory signaling system in multiple developing organ systems [1]. To date, the teratogenicity of exogenous cannabinoid exposure is not well understood. In animal models, early prenatal exposure before or during organogenesis or exposure to high cannabinoid doses (up to 60 mg/kg over a period of 1–3 months) resulted in neurotoxic effects in the hippocampus, amygdala, and cerebral cortex [9], with some animal models showing neurotoxicity comparable to fetal alcohol syndrome [2]. Of note, these studies investigated exposures much higher than typical human consumption.

While animal models raised concerns for teratogenic effects of exogenous cannabinoids, there has been little evidence to support gross developmental abnormalities in humans. The Generation R Study, a prospective study of 7452 mothers to investigate the impact of substance use during pregnancy on fetal growth, found maternal cannabis in early pregnancy (<18 weeks gestation) or continued use throughout pregnancy is associated with growth restriction in mid to late pregnancy and lower birth weight [15]. El Marrouin et al. also demonstrated a dose response, with no significant changes in birth weight among the children of occasional (monthly) cannabis-using women, significantly lower birth weight among children of moderate (weekly) cannabis-using women, and the lowest birth weights among heavy (daily) cannabis-using women. To further investigate the impact of maternal cannabis use on fetal growth and development, Hurd et al. characterized midgestational postmortem human fetuses [13]. Exposed fetuses had a significant reduction in foot length and body weight for gestational age, with fetal foot length negatively correlating with the amount and frequency of maternal cannabis use.

Cognitive Effects of Prenatal Cannabis Exposure

CB1R is highly expressed in striatal, limbic, and cortical regions that coordinate cognitive and emotional function [11]. Similarly, there is a high density of CB1R in the hippocampus, which is fundamental to memory acquisition, consolidation, and retrieval [9]. Specific brain regions impacted by prenatal cannabis exposure provide insights into the expected neurocognitive impacts (Box 4.2). For example, development of the prefrontal cortex appears particularly vulnerable to maternal cannabis use, resulting in disinhibition that may underly many of the cognitive deficits associated with long-term cannabis use. Reductions in cortical neuronal cell populations and decreased glutamatergic neurotransmission in newborn rats have also been observed in prenatal cannabis exposure, which may contribute to learning deficits and decreased emotional reactivity [16]. In the hippocampus, prenatal THC exposure disrupts neuronal migration, elongation of GABA-containing interneurons, and synaptogenesis, predicting impairments in memory and learning [1, 7]. Disruption of endocannabinoid signaling in the hippocampus and cortex (particularly the frontal lobe) predicts cognitive, memory, and neurobehavioral deficits [17].

Neurodevelopmental vulnerability to exogenous cannabinoid exposure is of particular concern during the perinatal period. Cannabinoids are lipophilic, readily cross the blood-brain barrier, and reach the brain of fetuses and newborns [2]. Approximately one-third of plasma THC undergoes cross-placental transfer during pregnancy [1, 4]. In utero cannabinoid exposure is associated with reorganization of neurotransmitter systems and cortical cell death and concurrent impairments in executive function, learning and memory, attention, visual perceptive tasks, and language comprehension and increased impulsivity and externalizing behavior [9, 17].

Multiple confounders, including comorbid tobacco and alcohol use, sociodemographic factors, and other psychological characteristics, have complicated studies of the neurodevelopmental consequences of maternal cannabis use during pregnancy. Most of the information on the developmental outcomes of prenatal cannabis exposure is derived from the Ottawa Prenatal Prospective Study (OPPS) and the Maternal Health Practices and Child Development Study (MHPCD), which followed the children of women who used cannabis, tobacco, and or alcohol from birth through adolescence [4]. The OPPS primarily enrolled low-risk Caucasian, middle class Canadian women to study prenatal exposure to tobacco and cannabis, whereas the MHPCD followed women generally of low socioeconomic status from Pittsburgh, approximately half of whom are Caucasian and half of whom are Black. The following sections will review key findings from the OPPS and MHPCD studies of the postnatal impact of maternal cannabis use during pregnancy through infancy, childhood, and adolescence (Fig. 4.2).

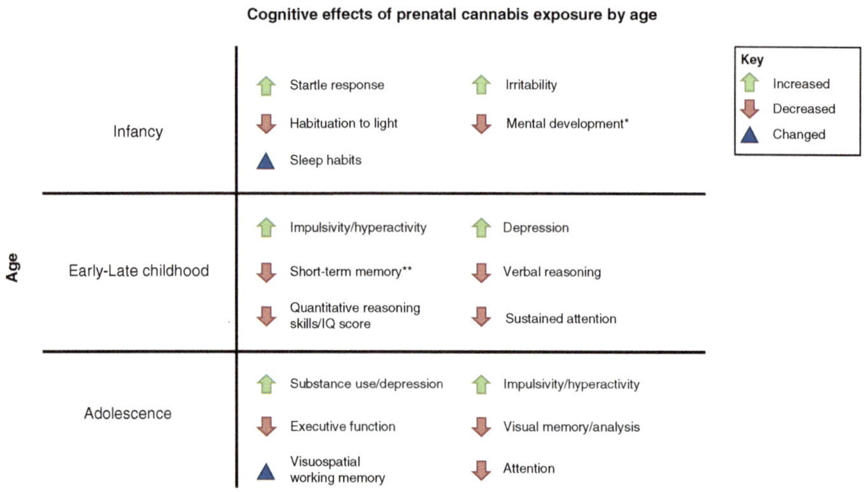

Fig. 4.2 The impact of prenatal cannabis exposure on neurocognition. This figure presents neurocognitive changes associated with prenatal cannabis exposure as reported in the MHPCD and OPPS longitudinal studies of maternal cannabis use. Findings are presented by age group: Infancy (birth to 3 years old), Early-Late childhood (3–13 years old), and Adolescence (14–22 years old). * Development changes were not present at 18 months of age in the MHPCD cohort and the OPPS did not report cognitive deficits between the ages of 1 and 3 years. ** Analysis by race between White and Black mothers shows disparities in effects of maternal cannabis use

Infancy

In neonates, prenatal cannabis exposure was strongly associated with increased startle response and a significant reduction in habituation to light, as well as altered sleep patterns and a trend toward increased irritability [4]. In the MHPCD cohort, using more than one joint per day in the third trimester was associated with decreased mental scores on the Bayley Scales of Infant Development at 9 months of age, which disappeared by 18 months old [4]. Similarly, the OPPS did not report cognitive deficits between the ages of 1 and 3 years, suggesting cognitive abnormalities are absent or subclinical in toddlers. In a third longitudinal study of prenatal cannabis exposure, Richardson et al. found use of one or more joints per day during the third trimester was associated with delayed mental development at 9 months of age [18].

Early Through Late Childhood

By age 3 years, first- or second-trimester cannabis exposure was associated with short-term memory (-1.1 IQ points/joint/day and -2.3 IQ points/joint/day, respectively) in the MHPCD cohort [19]. When analyzing the impact of prenatal cannabis use by race, a more complex interaction emerges. Among the children of Black mothers, there was a significant impact of first-trimester cannabis use on composite score (-0.9 IQ points/joint/day), short-term memory subscale (-1.1 IQ points/joint/day), and verbal reasoning (-1.5 IQ points/joint/day). Second-trimester use was also significantly associated with lower short-term memory subscores (-1.8 IQ points/joint/day). Interestingly, among the children of White mothers, there was no significant effect of prenatal cannabis use during any trimester of pregnancy on the composite IQ or subscale scores, which may be mediated or offset by participation in daycare or preschool. Similar to the main findings of the MHPCD study, in the OPPS study, smoking six or more joints a week (heavy exposure) during pregnancy was associated with decreases in verbal perceptual, general cognitive index, and memory domain scores of the McCarthy Scales of Children's Abilities at 4 years of age [20]. Thus, both studies support the impact of prenatal cannabis exposure cognitive functions including short-term memory and verbal reasoning in early childhood, though it is important to note other factors may mediate or confound the impact of exposure.

At age 5 years, in the OPPS cohort, prenatal cannabis exposure was associated with a dose-dependent trend in deficits of sustained attention, with the highest omission error rate in children of mothers who used more than six joints a week and the lowest omission error rate in children whose mothers used no more than one joint a week [21]. While heavy use mothers reported higher ratings on an impulsive/hyperactive scale, these differences were not statistically significant. In the MHPCD cohort, at age 6 years, heavy cannabis use (one or more joints a day) during the first or second trimester is associated with lower verbal reasoning scores [22]. Heavy cannabis use during the second trimester is also associated with deficits in short-term memory and during the second or third trimester is associated with decreased quantitative scores. In any trimester, heavy cannabis use is associated with lower composite score and quantitative reasoning. At age 10 years, heavy first- and third-trimester exposure (>0.89 joints/day) is associated with increased hyperactivity and impulsivity, and heavy second-trimester exposure is associated with increased impulsivity [23]. Heavy exposure is also associated with increased levels of depression and lower child IQ.

Adolescence

Synthesis of the findings from OPPS and MHPCD through adolescence shows prenatal cannabis exposure adversely impacts adolescent executive function, particularly attentional behavior and visual analysis and hypothesis testing, with impacts lasting through childhood [4]. By age 13–16 years, adolescents in the OPPS cohort with heavy cannabis exposure (>0.86 joints/day) exhibited deficits in visual memory, visual analysis, and ability to maintain attention [4]. Similarly, adolescents in the MHPCD cohort demonstrate deficits in visual analysis and impulse control aspects of executive functioning. A functional magnetic resonance imaging (fMRI) study of 18–22-year-old youth showed prenatal exposure is associated with alternations in neural activity during visuospatial working memory tasks [4]. Maternal cannabis use predicts earlier onset and increased frequency of substance use among adolescent children [7].

Cognitive Effects of Adolescent Cannabis Exposure

Similar to prenatal exposure, cannabis use by adolescents and young adults prior to completion of neurodevelopment poses an increased risk to the cognitive effects of cannabis use. The ECS continues to function as a modulator of neurodevelopment via regulation of synaptic pruning and signaling pathways, which facilitate learning, memory, appetite, and neuroprotection and modulate anxiety, depression, and pain [4]. Cannabis use impacts psychomotor speed, complex attention, planning and sequencing ability, executive function, and working memory [7]. Epidemiologic studies report adolescents with heavy cannabis use experience higher rates of depression and anxiety, a greater burden of psychotic symptoms, impairments in learning and memory, and deficits in executive functioning, including decision-making, processing speed, and attention [9]. Similarly, a review of studies of cognition demonstrates diminished performance on tasks requiring effortful performance, including executive functioning, verbal free recall, decision-making, abstract reasoning, and complex spatial work [24, 25].

While the literature investigating the cognitive effects of adolescent cannabis use is expanding, synthesis of evidence is limited by variable outcome measures, relatively small study sizes, and inconsistency in reporting the frequency or quantity of cannabis use between studies. Where available, frequency or quantity of cannabis use associated with reported neurologic changes or impairments will be noted. One of the most provocative findings was reported by Meier et al., who followed 1037 individuals from birth, with neuropsychological testing at 13 years and 38 years of age [26]. In this cohort, persistent cannabis use (at least 4 days per week) is associated with a greater decline in neuropsychological function assessed by full-scale IQ (WAIS-IV) of approximately eight points, as well as declines in verbal IQ, performance IQ, and multiple other subtests. Impairments were noted in executive function, memory, processing speed, perceptual reasoning, verbal comprehension, and verbal learning and recall. Of note, adolescent-onset cannabis users did not fully regain neuropsychological functioning with abstinence, supporting the neurotoxic effects of cannabis on the developing brain.

Subsequently, there has been a robust debate about the impact of cannabis use on IQ and interest in how this correlates with academic performance. Persistent cannabis use throughout high school is associated with lower grade point average (GPA) and scholastic aptitude test scores, though these observations were not significant after controlling for alcohol and tobacco use [25, 27]. One contributor of poorer academic performance may be externalizing and attention/concentration problems, which often co-occur with cannabis use [25].

To better understand the impact of cannabis use on neurodevelopment and cognition, Becker et al. conducted a prospective analysis of cannabis-using adolescents who used at least five times per week for at least 1 year, with onset of use before age 17 years [24]. Individuals were selected who were sober at the time of enrolment, effectively limiting the evaluation to the effects of chronic cannabis use. In these adolescents, there was decreased white matter growth in the central and parietal regions of the right and left superior longitudinal fasciculus, which is associated with diminished performance in verbal learning and memory [24, 25]. As described in the study, more "hits" or uses of cannabis are negatively associated with changes in white matter connectivity in a seemingly dose-dependent manner.

Similarly, in a second longitudinal study, Camchong et al. followed treatment-seeking adolescents with more than 50 lifetime "exposures to" (or uses of) cannabis who were sober at the time of study entry (29). In this cohort, decreased functional connectivity between caudal anterior cingulate cortex and superior frontal gyrus predicted higher amounts of cannabis use in the following months defined as number of days used. More frequent cannabis use also predicted lower intelligence quotient (IQ), though this was a nonsignificant trend when including alcohol as covariate, and slower cognitive function [25, 28]. The study authors propose one possible mechanism may be increased dopamine release in the anterior cingulate cortex, resulting in reciprocal downregulation of D2 receptor availability and subsequent impairment of cognitive functioning and decision-making.

The frequency of and the age of onset of cannabis use are also associated with a negative impact on working memory including recall time and sustained attention. In the Philadelphia Neurodevelopmental Cohort, adolescents who reported frequent cannabis use (more than three times per week) performed worse on measures of executive control compared to occasional cannabis users (twice per week or less) and non-using adolescents [29]. Earlier age of onset is associated with worse performance in occasional users, though this group exhibited better executive control, memory, and social cognition. In a study by Solowij et al., cannabis users (average 14 days of use per month) exhibited impaired verbal learning and memory over five study procedure trials, with impairment in learning, retention, and retrieval [30]. Younger age of onset, longer duration, and more frequent or higher quantity of cannabis use are all associated with fewer total words learned and recalled. Additionally, adolescents who use cannabis an average of 10 days per month show increased risky and impulsive decision makers, adopting strategies with higher levels of uncertainty and utilizing information less efficiently [31].

Similar to animal models, impairments in executive function associated with adolescent cannabis use are more persistent in abstinence when compared with adult cannabis users [9]. Earlier age of onset is associated with greater impairment in learning and memory, decision-making, attention, and other executive functions. Among adult users, those who began using prior to age 16 years show deficits in visual scanning, sustained attention, and working memory compared to late-onset and non-using adults [11]. In a study of adults who chronically use cannabis, onset in adolescence before age 15 years (mean use of 1.7 joints per day) is associated with poorer cognitive performance in executive functioning in adulthood [32]. Similarly, a second study demonstrated onset of use prior to age 16 years (average 24.8 smoking episodes and 14.8 g cannabis consumed per week) is associated with poorer cognitive performance on measures of executive function, with more difficulty inhibiting inappropriate responses and maintaining cognitive set [33]. In these individuals, earlier age of onset is positively correlated with changes in frontal white matter tracts as assessed by fractional anisotropy [34]. Taken together these findings suggest that impairments in executive function and cognition may result from adolescent cannabis use and persist into adulthood due to alterations in neurodevelopment.

Neuroimaging Studies of Adolescent Cannabis Use

Neuroimaging studies have identified mixed results regarding structural changes associated with adolescent cannabis use. For detailed reviews of neuroimaging findings please see Chye et al. [11]. Synthesis of neuroimaging studies is limited by small study size, heterogeneity of population and techniques, and multiple other confounders. Yet, two regions in which structural changes are often noted in cross-sectional and longitudinal structural and functional studies are the frontal lobe, particularly orbitofrontal cortex (OFC), and parietal lobes. Reduced frontal lobe thickness is also predictive of adolescent-onset cannabis use in adult users. As with cognitive impairments, earlier age of onset may be associated with the magnitude of structural change. However, changes in brain structure are not necessarily equivocal to functional changes. For example, another more consistent finding is smaller bilateral hippocampi in adolescents who use cannabis compared with non-using peers. One study found hippocampal volume is positively associated with verbal learning performance in adolescents who do not use cannabis, whereas it is not associated with verbal learning in cannabis-using adolescents, suggesting altered structure-functional relationship may underlie cognitive differences associated with adolescent cannabis use.

As imaging technologies have advanced, there has been more focus on evaluating white matter integrity and structure-functional relationships. Longitudinal studies suggest continued heavy cannabis use alters development of white matter microstructure and may contribute to functional impairments [24]. The most consistently implicated findings are poorer white matter integrity in the superior longitudinal fasciculus, the superior temporal gyrus, and the corpus callosum [11, 24]. Poorer white matter integrity has been reported in axon fibers encompassing the frontal lobe and bilateral hippocampi. Frontal and bilateral parietal lobe activation is also implicated in attention network task-based connectivity, with adolescent cannabis users showing greater activation and poorer task performance. This suggests adolescents who use cannabis may compensate with increased brain activation to mitigate functional impairment.

One notable limitation of neuroimaging studies is that the directionality of change is not known. In other words, it is not known if differences in neuroimaging result in behaviors that are associated with more frequent cannabis use or if cannabis use alters brain structure and connectivity. The Adolescent Brain Cognitive Development (ABCD) study (https://abcdstudy.org) is a multisite prospective longitudinal study now underway that may help to better understand the contribution of cannabis and other substance use, age of onset, and gender, among other biological and behavioral determinants, on neurodevelopmental trajectory.

Future Directions

Taken together, what is known about the role of the ECS in neurodevelopment and the impact of cannabinoid exposure during the prenatal and adolescent periods, findings suggest adolescence is a critical period of increased risk for adverse outcomes from cannabis use [9]. No amount of cannabis is known to be safe for the developing brain. However, much remains unknown. Very little is known about the impact of prenatal cannabinoid exposure and adolescent cannabis use on the ECS. Further, to date no studies have evaluated the effects of prenatal or adolescent cannabinoid exposure on endocannabinoid levels. Animal studies and clinical experience also suggest there may be notable differences between genders that are not well understood [10, 11]. Many of the studies completed to date are cross-sectional or retrospective and do not allow for adequate evaluation of confounders or causality [9]. Similarly, longitudinal studies have yet to be conducted to investigate the unprecedented increases in THC concentration and routes of administration as recreational cannabis is increasingly legalized and commercialized. The past decade of legalization has been predominantly driven by political processes. Medicine and science must now respond with evidence-based studies to better understand the impact these changes are having on youths' developing brains.

References

1. Harkany T, Guzman M, Galve-Roperh I, Berghuis P, Devi LA, Mackie K. The emerging functions of endocannabinoid signaling during CNS development. Trends Pharmacol Sci. 2007;28(2):83–92.
2. Fernandez-Ruiz J, Berrendero F, Hernandez ML, Ramos JA. The endogenous cannabinoid system and brain development. Trends Neurosci. 2000;23(1):14–20.
3. Lu HC, Mackie K. Review of the endocannabinoid system. Biol Psychiatry Cogn Neurosci Neuroimaging. 2021;6(6):607–15.
4. Wu CS, Jew CP, Lu HC. Lasting impacts of prenatal cannabis exposure and the role of endogenous cannabinoids in the developing brain. Future Neurol. 2011;6(4):459–80.
5. Bernard C, Milh M, Morozov YM, Ben-Ari Y, Freund TF, Gozlan H. Altering cannabinoid signaling during development disrupts neuronal activity. Proc Natl Acad Sci U S A. 2005;102(26):9388–93.
6. Harkany T, Mackie K, Doherty P. Wiring and firing neuronal networks: endocannabinoids take center stage. Curr Opin Neurobiol. 2008;18(3):338–45.
7. Jutras-Aswad D, DiNieri JA, Harkany T, Hurd YL. Neurobiological consequences of maternal cannabis on human fetal development and its neuropsychiatric outcome. Eur Arch Psychiatry Clin Neurosci. 2009;259(7):395–412.
8. Keimpema E, Barabas K, Morozov YM, Tortoriello G, Torii M, Cameron G, et al. Differential subcellular recruitment of monoacylglycerol lipase generates spatial specificity of 2-arachidonoyl glycerol signaling during axonal pathfinding. J Neurosci. 2010;30(42):13992–4007.
9. Lubman DI, Cheetham A, Yucel M. Cannabis and adolescent brain development. Pharmacol Ther. 2015;148:1–16.
10. Schneider M. Cannabis use in pregnancy and early life and its consequences: animal models. Eur Arch Psychiatry Clin Neurosci. 2009;259(7):383–93.
11. Chye Y, Christensen E, Yucel M. Cannabis use in adolescence: a review of neuroimaging findings. J Dual Diagn. 2020;16(1):83–105.
12. Gomez M, Hernandez M, Johansson B, de Miguel R, Ramos JA, Fernandez-Ruiz J. Prenatal cannabinoid and gene expression for neural adhesion molecule L1 in the fetal rat brain. Brain Res Dev Brain Res. 2003;147(1–2):201–7.
13. Hurd YL, Wang X, Anderson V, Beck O, Minkoff H, Dow-Edwards D. Marijuana impairs growth in mid-gestation fetuses. Neurotoxicol Teratol. 2005;27(2):221–9.
14. Wang X, Dow-Edwards D, Anderson V, Minkoff H, Hurd YL. Discrete opioid gene expression impairment in the human fetal brain associated with maternal marijuana use. Pharmacogenomics J. 2006;6(4):255–64.
15. El Marroun H, Tiemeier H, Steegers EA, Jaddoe VW, Hofman A, Verhulst FC, et al. Intrauterine cannabis exposure affects fetal growth trajectories: the generation R study. J Am Acad Child Adolesc Psychiatry. 2009;48(12):1173–81.
16. Antonelli T, Tomasini MC, Tattoli M, Cassano T, Tanganelli S, Finetti S, et al. Prenatal exposure to the CB1 receptor agonist WIN 55,212-2 causes learning disruption associated with impaired cortical NMDA receptor function and emotional reactivity changes in rat offspring. Cereb Cortex. 2005;15(12):2013–20.
17. Wang X, Dow-Edwards D, Keller E, Hurd YL. Preferential limbic expression of the cannabinoid receptor mRNA in the human fetal brain. Neuroscience. 2003;118(3):681–94.
18. Richardson GA, Day NL, Goldschmidt L. Prenatal alcohol, marijuana, and tobacco use: infant mental and motor development. Neurotoxicol Teratol. 1995;17(4):479–87.
19. Day NL, Richardson GA, Goldschmidt L, Robles N, Taylor PM, Stoffer DS, et al. Effect of prenatal marijuana exposure on the cognitive development of offspring at age three. Neurotoxicol Teratol. 1994;16(2):169–75.
20. Fried PA, Watkinson B. 36- and 48-month neurobehavioral follow-up of children prenatally exposed to marijuana, cigarettes, and alcohol. J Dev Behav Pediatr. 1990;11(2):49–58.

21. Fried PA, Watkinson B, Gray R. A follow-up study of attentional behavior in 6-year-old children exposed prenatally to marihuana, cigarettes, and alcohol. Neurotoxicol Teratol. 1992;14(5):299–311.
22. Goldschmidt L, Richardson GA, Willford J, Day NL. Prenatal marijuana exposure and intelligence test performance at age 6. J Am Acad Child Adolesc Psychiatry. 2008;47(3):254–63.
23. Day NL, Leech SL, Goldschmidt L. The effects of prenatal marijuana exposure on delinquent behaviors are mediated by measures of neurocognitive functioning. Neurotoxicol Teratol. 2011;33(1):129–36.
24. Becker MP, Collins PF, Lim KO, Muetzel RL, Luciana M. Longitudinal changes in white matter microstructure after heavy cannabis use. Dev Cogn Neurosci. 2015;16:23–35.
25. Cyrus E, Coudray MS, Kiplagat S, Mariano Y, Noel I, Galea JT, et al. A review investigating the relationship between cannabis use and adolescent cognitive functioning. Curr Opin Psychol. 2020;38:38–48.
26. Meier MH, Caspi A, Ambler A, Harrington H, Houts R, Keefe RS, et al. Persistent cannabis users show neuropsychological decline from childhood to midlife. Proc Natl Acad Sci U S A. 2012;109(40):E2657–64.
27. Meier MH, Hill ML, Small PJ, Luthar SS. Associations of adolescent cannabis use with academic performance and mental health: A longitudinal study of upper middle class youth. Drug Alcohol Depend. 2015;156:207–12.
28. Camchong J, Lim KO, Kumra S. Adverse Effects of Cannabis on Adolescent Brain Development: A Longitudinal Study. Cereb Cortex. 2017;27(3):1922–30.
29. Scott JC, Wolf DH, Calkins ME, Bach EC, Weidner J, Ruparel K, et al. Cognitive functioning of adolescent and young adult cannabis users in the Philadelphia Neurodevelopmental Cohort. Psychol Addict Behav. 2017;31(4):423–34.
30. Solowij N, Jones KA, Rozman ME, Davis SM, Ciarrochi J, Heaven PCL, et al. Verbal learning and memory in adolescent cannabis users, alcohol users and non-users. Psychopharmacology. 2011;216(1):131–44.
31. Solowij N, Jones KA, Rozman ME, Davis SM, Ciarrochi J, Heaven PC, et al. Reflection impulsivity in adolescent cannabis users: a comparison with alcohol-using and non-substance-using adolescents. Psychopharmacology (Berl). 2012;219(2):575–86.
32. Fontes MA, Bolla KI, Cunha PJ, Almeida PP, Jungerman F, Laranjeira RR, et al. Cannabis use before age 15 and subsequent executive functioning. Br J Psychiatry. 2011;198(6):442–7.
33. Gruber SA, Sagar KA, Dahlgren MK, Racine M, Lukas SE. Age of onset of marijuana use and executive function. Psychol Addict Behav. 2012;26(3):496–506.
34. Gruber SA, Silveri MM, Dahlgren MK, Yurgelun-Todd D. Why so impulsive? White matter alterations are associated with impulsivity in chronic marijuana smokers. Exp Clin Psychopharmacol. 2011;19(3):231–42.

What Clinicians Need to Know About Adolescent Cannabis Use in Outpatient Mental Health Settings

5

Paula Riggs

Case

Johnny D. is a 17-year-old male with a history of attention deficit hyperactivity disorder (ADHD), combined type, referred by his pediatrician to an outpatient psychiatry clinic for evaluation and treatment of worsening anxiety, "lack of motivation, and worsening academic performance since the beginning of the school year". During an initial interview with Johnny and his mother, Johnny's mother reported that his grades have dropped from a "B" average to C's and D's during the current school year. She added, "he just doesn't seem to care much about school or anything else, lately since he started hanging out with a new group of friends this year". She said the school safety officer caught Johnny and three of his new friends skipping class and "vaping" in the school parking lot. All were ticketed, suspended from school for a week, and required to attend weekend drug and alcohol classes. She adds, "He's totally lost interest in playing football, his grades have dropped, I can't get him to his chores around the house, and he stays out after curfew. To top it all off, he sold the coin collection his grandfather gave him to get money to buy weed."

During a subsequent clinical interview with Johnny alone, he reported that he started "vaping" nicotine after he and his mother moved to Colorado last summer. When school started, he started "vaping" nicotine and cannabis "pretty much every day" over the past 8 months. He said that marijuana initially helped him feel less "stressed out," adding that he's not sure it's working as well as it used to. He said that he's had to increase his use from once or twice per day to "several" times per

P. Riggs (✉)
Department of Psychiatry, University of Colorado School of Medicine, Aurora, CO, USA
e-mail: paula.riggs@cuanschutz.edu

P. Riggs, T. Thant (eds.), *Cannabis in Psychiatric Practice*, Psychiatry Update 3,
https://doi.org/10.1007/978-3-031-04874-6_5

day in the past few months in order to "get the same chill." He agrees that the escalation in his cannabis and nicotine use has "kind of become a problem," but he's not sure what he wants to do about it. He adds, "I don't really know what life would be like without it now."

Introduction

Many aspects of this case will be familiar to behavioral health clinicians working in outpatient mental health settings. Adolescents often seek mental health treatment for symptoms of ADHD, depression, or anxiety. As in Johnny's case, affiliation with a new substance-involved peer group can lead to initiation of cannabis use which can rapidly progress to more frequent habitual pattern of use that suggests an evolving cannabis use disorder (CUD). Johnny's case also illustrates how escalation to daily or near daily cannabis use may lead to worsening academic performance and a loss of interest in previously enjoyed activities. Parents often observe decreased motivation and an increase in "moodiness," irritability, and "sneaky" behavior. The history provided by both Johnny and his mother suggests that he is likely to meet criteria for at least a moderately severe cannabis use disorder (CUD) based on their endorsement of the following four of eleven diagnostic criteria from the *Diagnostic and Statistical Manual of Mental Disorders, Fifth Edition* (DSM 5) [1]: (a) continued use despite persistent or recurring social or interpersonal consequences; (b) recurrent use resulting in a failure to fulfill role obligations at school/home; (c) important social, occupational, or recreational activities given up or reduced; (d) tolerance (increased amount to achieve same effect or diminished effect with same amount). In a confidential clinical interview with the adolescent alone (without parent/guardian), additional history should be elicited to determine whether Johnny meets criteria for any of the additional seven DSM 5 diagnostic criteria for cannabis use disorder. He should also be asked about his previous and current use of alcohol and other drugs. Based on his history of daily nicotine use, Johnny is also likely to meet diagnostic criteria for nicotine use disorder. Co-use of both nicotine and cannabis has become increasingly common among adolescents in the context of an ever-expanding legalized cannabis environment in the U.S. Recent studies indicate that among adolescents who report regular vaping, co-use of nicotine and cannabis is more common than the use of nicotine or cannabis alone [2]. Vaping is one of the most common ways adolescents in the U.S. currently use marijuana and nicotine. The 2020 Monitoring the Future (MTF) Survey indicates that the prevalence of past-year marijuana vaping among eighth, 10th, and 12th grade high school students is 8.1%, 19.1%, and 22.1%, respectively. The prevalence of daily or near daily marijuana vaping is 0.7%, 1.7%, and 2.5%, respectively [3]. The prevalence of past-year nicotine vaping is 16.6%, 30.7%, and 34.5%, respectively and daily/near daily nicotine vaping is 2%, 5.6%, and 8.6%, respectively [3].

The impact of an expanding cannabis legalized environment in the U.S. on trends in youth cannabis use is not yet clear and research findings are mixed. The national prevalence of marijuana use among youth increased rapidly, between 2008 and 2011, surpassing tobacco use. During this period past-year marijuana use increased 31%, past month use increased 42%, and heavy monthly marijuana use (20 or more times) increased 80%, from 5% in 2008 to 9% in 2011 [4]. Increased use was associated with a concomitant decrease in the perceived harms of cannabis use and a growing acceptance of cannabis use as normalized behavior [4]. As the number of states with legalized cannabis has steadily increased since 2009, national surveys have not shown a significant increase in adolescent marijuana use [5, 6]. However, it is important to note that the states legalizing medical marijuana after 2008 had a higher prevalence of adolescent marijuana use and lower perception of risk prior to legalization during the period between 2002 and 2008. Although legalization has not driven an increase in youth prevalence, both Colorado and Washington states have reported a significant increase in marijuana-related hospitalizations, emergency department and urgent care visits (e.g., hyperemesis, psychosis, inadvertent exposures), suicides, and motor vehicle accidents. The potency of cannabis products sold in legalized commercial markets has risen dramatically since 2011. High potency concentrates (e.g., "dabs," "wax," "shatter"), containing 70–95% THC, currently occupy about 25% of the market share of commercial cannabis products sold in the U.S. Higher potency is associated with greater abuse liability and significantly greater risk of psychosis, especially in adolescents and young adults [7, 8].

A substantial body of research indicates that adolescents are more vulnerable to addiction and mental health problems due to rapid brain development and synaptic pruning that occurs from about age 10 throughout adolescence into young adulthood [9]. Regular cannabis use during adolescence interferes with the role of the endocannabinoid system in regulating mood and reward as well as development of the prefrontal cortex [10]. Regular marijuana use before age 18 at least quadruples the risk of psychosis, doubles the risk of developing a depressive or anxiety disorder by young adulthood, increases the risk of addiction to other substances tried later, and is associated with persistent neurocognitive deficits and reductions in adult IQ that may not be fully reversible even with abstinence [9, 10]. Current research suggests that the frequency of marijuana use during adolescence is associated with poorer psychosocial outcomes in a dose-related fashion. Adolescents who use marijuana regularly are less likely to finish high school or obtain a college degree and more likely to be unemployed or underemployed, welfare dependent, and have lower overall life satisfaction compared to non-using peers. More research is needed to disentangle the extent to which marijuana use directly contributes to these outcomes or whether other factors independently predispose individuals to both marijuana use and negative psychosocial outcomes. Marijuana has also been associated with an *amotivational syndrome*, defined as a diminished or absent drive to engage in typically rewarding activities as evidenced in the case presented at the beginning of this chapter. Results of several recent studies suggest an association between marijuana use and suicidal thoughts and attempted suicide among teens [9]. However, it is not yet clear whether the association between cannabis use and suicidality, if confirmed, is directly related to cannabis use or other antecedent factors common to both. The short-term effects and longer-term negative impact of adolescent cannabis use on neurocognitive development, risk of psychosis, and poorer psychosocial outcomes underscore the important role of clinicians working in outpatient mental health settings in substance prevention, screening, early intervention, and treatment (Highlights Box 5.1).

Substance Screening and Clinical Evaluation

In outpatient mental health settings, adolescents like Johnny often present for treatment of depression, anxiety, ADHD, or other psychiatric disorders. Unless clinicians working in these settings systematically screen for substance use, substance use may not be discovered until treatment for other mental health problems is well underway. Ample research shows that children and adolescents with mental health problems are at increased risk for developing or having a co-occurring substance use disorder (SUD) compared to youth in the general population [9]. Substance use complicates the treatment and clinical management of pre-existing psychiatric disorders and increases the risk of developing new psychiatric symptoms and other mental health problems [9]. For these reasons, routine substance screening is recommended for all youth ages 12 and older in pediatric primary care and outpatient mental health settings.

There are a number of validated brief substance screening measures. Two of the most commonly used measures used to assess risk in adolescents ages 12–17 are the Brief Screener for Tobacco, Alcohol, and other Drugs (BSTAD) and the Screening to Brief Intervention (S2BI). Both can be administered online and take less than 2 min to complete. The BSTAD uses highly sensitive and specific cutoffs to identify various SUDs among adolescents 12–17 years of age [17]. The S2BI uses a stem question: "How many times in the past year have you used" tobacco/nicotine (including vaping); alcohol, marijuana, illicit drugs (e.g., cocaine, methamphetamine); prescription medications not prescribed to you (Adderall, pain medications); inhalants and synthetic drugs (e.g., K2, spice, kratom). Response frequencies for each drug category are "never," "once or twice," "monthly," and "weekly or more." Adolescents who report using "once or twice" in the past year are not likely to meet diagnostic criteria for a SUD. Teens who report using at least "monthly" are likely to have a mild-moderate SUD and those using "weekly or more" are likely to have a moderate-severe SUD, based on DSM 5 criteria.

Both the BSTAD and S2BI are designed to be self- or clinician-administered. However, in outpatient settings, self-administered screening information may get "buried" among an array of clinic intake forms that patients and parents are asked to complete prior to an initial clinical evaluation. Whether self- or clinician-administered, it is important for clinicians to administer or review substance screening responses during an initial clinical evaluation. This should be done in the context of a confidential interview with the adolescent alone (without parent/guardian). Ideally, screening results should be scored, interpreted, and discussed with the adolescent in the same visit using a nonjudgmental, motivational interviewing approach. For example, if Johnny had reported "no use" in the past year, the clinician should positively reinforce or congratulate them for "healthy decision making" and provide relevant research-based psychoeducation about the risks associated with adolescent drug and alcohol use (see Highlights Box 5.2 psychoeducation resources). Teens who report using "once or twice" in the past year are not likely to meet DSM 5 diagnostic criteria for a SUD. For such youth, brief medically based advice and psychoeducation about the risks associated with drug/alcohol use during adolescence may help prevent progression to more regular substance use or SUD. Adolescents who report using "monthly" are likely to have a mild-moderate SUD and should be further evaluated using DSM 5 diagnostic criteria to determine SUD diagnosis and severity. If mild-moderate SUD is confirmed, psychoeducation and brief intervention using motivational enhancement may be an appropriate next step for such youth if the clinician has brief intervention training and experience. Adolescents like Johnny who report using "weekly or more" are likely to meet DSM 5 diagnostic criteria for a moderate-severe SUD. If DSM 5 SUD diagnosis is confirmed and the clinician is not dually trained to provide evidence-based substance treatment, the youth should be referred for a more comprehensive subspecialty substance evaluation and treatment if clinically indicated.

If the outpatient mental health setting does not have co-located subspecialty substance treatment services, such youth should be referred to evidence-based subspecialty substance treatment using motivational enhancement and a "warm handoff" approach to facilitate substance treatment engagement. A "warm handoff" can be facilitated by establishing a formal referral relationship with one or more substance treatment providers/programs offering evidence-based substance treatment followed by collaborative development of a coordinated care model between mental health and substance treatment providers if services are not co-located. Despite the challenges, the referring psychiatrist or behavioral health clinician should make every effort to coordinate care with the substance treatment provider and continue to provide ongoing treatment for co-occurring psychiatric disorders while the patient is enrolled in substance treatment. Mental health clinicians and substance treatment providers should also collaboratively plan and coordinate and individually tailor continuity of care to address a patient's ongoing psychiatric/mental health treatment and recovery support services as clinically indicated. A recent Charting Pediatrics podcast provides a more detailed explanation and example of a "warm handoff" that enhances substance treatment engagement among referred youth.

Treatment for Cannabis Use Disorder

There are a number of family-based, group, and individual treatment interventions with proven efficacy for adolescents and young adults with SUD. However, there is considerable clinical and research consensus that the most effective current treatment for cannabis use disorder is motivational enhancement therapy (MET) +

cognitive-behavioral therapy (CBT) + contingency management (CM). MET is a systematic form of intervention designed to produce rapid, internally motivated change; the therapy does not attempt to treat the person, but rather mobilize his or her own internal resources for change and engagement in treatment. CBT is a form of psychotherapy that teaches people strategies to identify and correct problematic behaviors in order to enhance self-control, stop drug use, and address a range of other problems that often co-occur with them. CM is a therapeutic management approach based on the principles of behavioral reinforcement which involves frequent monitoring of the target behavior and the provision (or removal) of tangible, positive rewards when the target behavior occurs (or does not).

Currently, there are no FDA-approved medications for the treatment of marijuana use disorder in adolescents, but research is active in this area. Agents being studied include the nutritional supplement N-acetylcysteine and chemicals called FAAH inhibitors, which may reduce withdrawal by inhibiting the breakdown of the body's own cannabinoids. Future directions include the study of substances called *allosteric modulators* that interact with cannabinoid receptors to inhibit THC's rewarding effects.

Integrated Treatment and Coordinated Care for Youth with Co-occurring Psychiatric and Substance Use Disorders

The majority of adolescents and young adults with cannabis and other SUD have at least one co-occurring psychiatric disorder, and there is considerable consensus among researchers and clinicians that treatment for individuals with co-occurring substance and psychiatric disorders should be integrated or concurrent and ideally provided by the same clinicians, program, or agency. However, in clinical settings where this is not possible, it is advisable to make every effort to coordinate psychiatric care with a subspecialty addiction treatment provider. There are a number of published guidelines that may be useful in developing models of coordinated care including a recently published evidence-based resource guide published by SAMHSA: *Treatment Considerations for Youth and Young Adults with Serious Emotional disturbances and Serious Mental Illnesses and Co-occurring Substance Use.*

Summary and Conclusion

Over the past decade, the expanding legalized cannabis environment and increased use of high potency cannabis in adolescents underscore the critical role of behavioral health clinicians as frontline first responders with regard to early identification and intervention in at risk youth and preventing progression to more serious substance involvement in youth who have initiated cannabis and/or other substances use. In order to be effective in this role, behavioral health clinicians working in outpatient mental health settings need to be familiar with valid substance screening tools, research-based psychoeducation resources, and have training and experience in motivational interviewing and brief interventions and develop "warm handoff" procedures for referring youth to subspecialty substance treatment providers using a collaborative coordinated care model.

Highlights Box 5.1 Key Points for Patient Psychoeducation

- Cannabis is addictive. An estimated 17% of youth who use marijuana develop cannabis use disorder (CUD) and onset before age 16 predicts 3× greater risk of CUD.
- Regular cannabis use before age 18 at least quadruples the risk of psychosis, doubles the risk of developing a depressive or anxiety disorder by young adulthood, increases the risk of addiction to other substances tried later, and is associated with persistent neurocognitive deficits and reductions in adult IQ that may not be fully reversible even with abstinence.
- High potency cannabis concentrates (e.g., dabs, wax, shatter) containing 75–95% THC have greater abuse liability and are associated with significantly increased risk of psychosis. There is a dose relationship between the frequency of cannabis use during adolescence and poorer psychosocial outcomes.
- Regular cannabis use before age 17 is associated with increased risk of suicidality and at least doubles the risk of developing an anxiety disorder by young adulthood.

Highlights Box 5.2 Key Points in Treatment and Management

Clinicians working in outpatient mental health settings should:

- Provide research-based psychoeducation to youth and families about the health and neurodevelopmental risks associated with adolescent cannabis use (e.g., "marijuana facts for teens"; "marijuana: What parents need to know" www.drugabuse.gov).
- Be familiar with valid brief substance screening tools (e.g., S2BI, BSTAD) and regularly screen youth ages 12 and older for cannabis and other substance use disorders.
- Know how to use motivational enhancement approaches for delivering "brief advice" and "brief interventions" and take advantage of the many online SBIRT training resources.
- Be familiar with subspecialty substance treatment programs providing evidence-based substance treatment and collaboratively develop "warm handoff" referral procedures using motivational enhancement to facilitate substance treatment engagement.
- Collaboratively develop ways to coordinate clinical care and concurrent treatment for co-occurring psychiatric and substance use disorders with substance treatment providers to whom youth are referred.

References

1. American Psychiatric Association. Diagnostic and statistical manual of mental disorders. 5th ed. Arlington, VA: American Psychiatric Association; 2013.
2. Lanza HI, Barrington-Trimis JL, McConnell R, Cho J, Braymiller JL, Krueger EA, et al. Trajectories of nicotine and cannabis vaping and polyuse from adolescence to young adulthood. JAMA Netw Open. 2020;3(10):e2019181-e. https://doi.org/10.1001/jamanetworkopen.2020.19181.
3. Johnston LD, Miech RA, O'Malley PM, Bachman JG, Schulenberg JE, Patrick ME. Monitoring the future national survey results on drug use, 1975–2020: overview, key findings on adolescent drug use. Ann Arbor, MI: Institute for Social Research, University of Michigan; 2021.
4. The Partnership at Drugfree.org, MetLife Foundation. The partnership attitude tracking study. 2011 parents and teens full report. 2011. https://drugfree.org/wp-content/uploads/2012/05/PATS-FULL-Report-FINAL-May-2-PDF-.pdf. Accessed 21 May 2021.
5. Ladegard K, Thurstone C, Rylander M. Marijuana legalization and youth. Pediatrics. 2020;145(Suppl 2):S165–S74. https://doi.org/10.1542/peds.2019-2056d.
6. Pacula RL, Smart R. Medical marijuana and marijuana legalization. Annu Rev Clin Psychol. 2017;13:397–419. https://doi.org/10.1146/annurev-clinpsy-032816-045128.
7. Murray RM, Quigley H, Quattrone D, Englund A, Di Forti M. Traditional marijuana, high-potency cannabis and synthetic cannabinoids: increasing risk for psychosis. World Psychiatry. 2016;15(3):195–204. https://doi.org/10.1002/wps.20341.
8. ElSohly MA, Mehmedic Z, Foster S, Gon C, Chandra S, Church JC. Changes in cannabis potency over the last 2 decades (1995-2014): analysis of current data in the United States. Biol Psychiatry. 2016;79(7):613–9. https://doi.org/10.1016/j.biopsych.2016.01.004.
9. National Institute on Drug Abuse. Marijuana research report. 2020. https://www.drugabuse.gov/download/1380/marijuana-research-report.pdf?v=d9e67cbd412ae5f340206c1a0d9c2bfd. Accessed 21 May 2021.
10. Leadbeater BJ, Ames ME, Linden-Carmichael AN. Age-varying effects of cannabis use frequency and disorder on symptoms of psychosis, depression and anxiety in adolescents and adults. Addiction. 2019;114(2):278–93.

Cannabis in the Child and Adolescent Emergency and Inpatient Psychiatric Settings

6

Gautam Rajendran and Thida Thant

Clinical Case

Bob was a 15-year-old male who was brought to the hospital when he was apprehended by the police while driving recklessly in a residential neighborhood. He had been cited a week earlier by the police for digging a large hole in his old school playground with a bizarre explanation about "digging up his past." On interview in the inpatient unit, he was quite paranoid about being watched on cameras and refused to take any medication and demanded discharge. He then became aggressive—first threatening and then assaulting staff when his request to be discharged was declined. He later suspected his parents of colluding with the treatment team (paranoia) to keep him in the hospital and was often staring into other patients' rooms, sometimes seated in the hallway for hours in one spot—claiming that he was using his "brain waves" to heal other patients (grandiosity, delusions). His refusal of medication and disruptive behavior in the milieu necessitated him being on a short-term certification and involuntary medication. His collateral history was notable for Bob being a fairly good student through middle school, with his use of cannabis starting at the age of 13. He started using concentrated forms of THC in the form of "wax and shatter" in the month prior to admission. Two weeks into his admission, on medication, Bob remained delusional and grandiose, reporting that he worked at a secret dispensary making "thousands" with plans to imminently open one of his own to market his cannabis products, and create "concentrates with up to 90% THC" levels. Bob's medical workup revealed normal blood counts, a normal metabolic panel, normal thyroid function, and a urine toxicology screen positive for

G. Rajendran (✉)
Children's Hospital Colorado, Aurora, CO, USA
e-mail: Gautam.Rajendran@childrenscolorado.org

T. Thant
Department of Psychiatry, University of Colorado School of Medicine, Aurora, CO, USA
e-mail: Thida.thant@cuanschutz.edu

P. Riggs, T. Thant (eds.), *Cannabis in Psychiatric Practice*, Psychiatry Update 3,
https://doi.org/10.1007/978-3-031-04874-6_6

cannabinoids and benzodiazepines (the latter most likely due to medication given by ambulance staff to manage his agitation). He did not have any fever, headache, signs of systemic infection, or focal neurological deficits to warrant neurological imaging or other invasive tests.

Introduction and Literature Reviewwe

Adolescent cannabis use complicates the clinical management of pre-existing psychiatric disorders and adds complexity to considerations of differential diagnosis. There is substantial evidence that cannabis use during adolescence increases the risk of suicidal ideation and behaviors and doubles the risk of developing depression and/or anxiety disorders. Multiple studies have also shown that adolescent-onset cannabis use at least quadruples the risk of initial-onset psychosis. However, the relationship between cannabis-induced psychosis and schizophrenia is less clear [1]. Based on clinical experience and an associated study in a tertiary care children's hospital in Colorado, the most common cannabis-associated reasons for inpatient psychiatric hospitalization are psychosis and severe depression with suicidality [2].

Psychotic Disorders

There is substantial research suggesting that cannabis use during adolescence significantly increases the risk of first-onset psychosis. Compared to non-cannabis using adolescents, risk of psychosis is higher in cannabis using youth, and this risk is even greater in those who have a genetic vulnerability or familial risk of schizophrenia [1, 3]. Starzer et al. [4] found that 32.2% of patients with a substance-induced psychosis converted to either bipolar or schizophrenia spectrum disorders. The highest conversion rate was found for cannabis-induced psychosis, with 47.4% converting to either schizophrenia or bipolar disorder within three to 5 years, respectively, after the initial onset of a cannabis-induced psychosis.

Taken together, the body of current research suggests that adolescent-onset cannabis use may precipitate earlier onset of schizophrenia in genetically vulnerable individuals and earlier onset is associated with a more severe and chronic course of illness and poorer prognosis [5, 6]. However, a growing body of research also indicates that adolescent-onset cannabis use can precipitate psychosis in youth without risk factors for schizophrenia [7, 8].

A study of more than 45,000 Swedish military conscripts showed a strong dose relationship effect of cannabis use at enrollment, and incidence of psychosis later in life [9]. In a study of over 100 subjects—the Dunedin birth cohort—individuals with cannabis use at age 15 and 18 had higher rates of both psychotic symptoms and schizophrenia at age 26 [10].

Di Forti et al. [11] reported that cases of first episode psychosis were much more likely to be current daily users (OR = 6.4) and to have smoked cannabis for more than 5 years (OR = 2.1). Among those who used cannabis, 78% of the cases group used high-potency cannabis (sinsemilla, "skunk") compared with 37% of the control group (OR 6.8). Di Forti et al. [12] and Gage et al. [13] reported that the regular use of cannabis as well as high-potency cannabis is linked to the development of psychotic disorders. Moore et al. [14] had also demonstrated a dose-response effect related to the frequency of cannabis use in adolescent-onset psychosis.

Compared to non-cannabis-related psychosis, some studies suggest that cannabis-induced psychosis may be less responsive to antipsychotic medications but more likely to remit within 12 months after cannabis cessation [15]. However, among adolescents who continue to use cannabis after the onset of a psychotic episode, psychosis is more likely to persist and develop into a chronic psychotic disorder.

Cannabis use also impacts the treatment course of patients with psychotic symptoms. D'Souza et al. reported an increase in psychotic symptoms in patients who had been stabilized on antipsychotic medication [16].

These findings underscore the clinical importance of making every effort to engage such youth in evidence-based substance treatment prior to or soon after discharge from inpatient hospitalization (further details in Chap. 5).

Mood and Anxiety Disorders

Current research suggest a bidirectional relationship between depression, anxiety disorders, and adolescent-onset cannabis use [17–19]. For example, a study by Hooshmand and colleagues followed more than 4000 adolescents from grades 9 to 12. Youth who reported more depressive symptoms in ninth grade were significantly more likely to smoke cigarettes and use cannabis by 12th grade and faster progression compared to those who reported few or no depression symptoms in ninth grade [20]. There is also growing evidence that the onset of regular cannabis use before age 18 significantly increases the risk of developing suicidality and major depressive disorder [21].

Several epidemiological studies have shown that chronic exposure to THC during adolescence is linked to depression and suicidality, especially at higher doses. In an Australian study, Silins et al. demonstrated an association between cannabis use and depressive symptoms, suicidality, and poor academic outcomes [22]. The link between cannabis use in adolescence and suicidality has been explored by Gobbi et al. in a meta-analysis including 11 studies comprising 23,317 individuals. Included studies used at least one assessment point under the age of 18, with a follow-up period to determine depression and suicidality from age 18 to 32 years (young adulthood) [23]. The investigators noted an odds ratio of 1.37 (95%CI) for developing depression in cannabis users in young adulthood compared to non-users. The pooled odds ratio was 1.50 for suicidal ideation and 3.46 for suicide attempts (both 95% CI). Carvalho et al. studies the association of adolescent cannabis use and suicidality in lower- and middle-income countries in 86,254 adolescents with a mean age of 13.7 years from 21 countries, assessing the suicide attempt in the past year and cannabis use in the past month and lifetime [24]. They noted that past 30-day cannabis use was significantly associated with suicide attempts (odds ratio 2.03; 85%CI) and lifetime cannabis use was also independently associated with suicide attempts (odds ratio 2.30; 95%CI).

In another study of Canadian subjects 15 and older, there were significant sex differences in the strength of the association between cannabis use and suicidal thoughts and attempts, but not regarding a Major Depressive Episode [25]. Females who reported using regularly (defined as more than once per week) reported higher levels of psychological distress and were more likely to report suicidal thoughts and attempts. In Colombia (Adalberto AC et al. 2020), in a study of 13- to 17-year-old high school students (n = 1462, mean age was 14.4 years), the lifetime prevalence of cannabis use was 11.6% and its consumption was associated with high suicide risk adjusted for other variables (OR = 1.88; 95%CI) [26].

Researchers have also replicated the neurobiological effects of cannabis on depression in animal models—with exposure to THC during adolescence increasing anhedonia and anxiety-related behavior paralleled by a decrease in serotonin activity. In human studies, cannabis has been noted to produce a transient amotivational state in occasional users [27] and a diminished response in the parietal and temporal cortices during reward activities [28].

Management of Psychotic and Mood Disorders Associated with Cannabis Abuse

The treatment considerations in patients who present with an acute onset of psychosis do not differ very much from the management of those with a chronic prodrome—apart from the need for frequent or urgent use of medication to manage agitation and aggression. However, with the increasing availability of cannabis and the prevalence of its use in high school age students—estimated at 23% in the past year [29]—the psychiatrist is often presented with a challenge of identifying the possibility of a substance-induced mood disorder. It is, nevertheless, important to try to distinguish a primary psychotic disorder from a substance-induced psychotic disorder during the inpatient stay for the purpose of family counseling and prognostication.

The patient with a more classical onset or primary psychosis is more likely to have

- A longer prodrome characterized by gradual social withdrawal.
- Unusual or overly focused interests and reduction in self-care over a period of months.
- A family history of psychotic disorders.
- Bizarre, detailed or complex delusions in patients who are using cannabis that seem out of proportion to cannabis use.

- Limited access to illicit substances due to their self-imposed limitation on socialization and paranoia towards others.
- An on-off pattern of cannabis use with longer periods of abstinence rather than continuing/escalating use.

Adolescents who have a substance-induced psychotic disorder often deny or show a complete lack of understanding of how substances might have induced a change in their behavior. This is especially true with those using synthetic or high-potency cannabinoids or those who are acutely intoxicated. Their family members and peers also describe an abrupt change in personality or behavior over a matter of days rather than months. They may also be much more resistant to taking psychometric or psychological tests aimed at assessing their mental status as opposed to those with an intrinsic or native psychosis who, because of partial insight in the early stages, are more open to assessment to understand their symptoms or their subjective experience of psychosis. Such patients, with a more native than substance-induced psychosis, might also be more prone to describe their use of substances like cannabis as an effort to manage their experiences or symptoms and be less evasive regarding their use.

Enquiries should also be made as to the content of their living habitat—as parents and caregivers are often able to provide information about clues to the form of cannabis consumed, such as residues in pipes in the case of resin, wrapping or packaging in the case of edibles, and concentrates in the form of vape products. Often there is indirect evidence of acquisition of cannabis concentrates in the form of electronic transactions for such product purchases.

In the case of the patient Bob, his initial medical workup including a complete blood count and metabolic panel (including liver function tests), thyroid panel, and fasting lipid panel was within normal limits. Laboratory workup was positive for cannabinoids and benzodiazepines (likely due to Lorazepam administered by emergency medical response staff to manage aggression).

Due to his florid psychotic symptoms and risk of physical aggression, he was started initially on Risperidone at a dose of 1 mg and this was titrated to 4 mg/day with minimal to no response. He needed frequent dosing of up to 2 mg of Lorazepam orally and intramuscularly additionally (up to a total of 6 mg/day) to manage his aggression. Bob was unable to tolerate Risperidone and noted to develop extrapyramidal symptoms such as cog wheel rigidity in his arms and a shuffling gait with poor balance. His further up-titration of Risperidone was limited by these extrapyramidal symptoms and the development of dystonia, which was treated using oral Benztropine. After 9 days on Risperidone, he was transitioned to Olanzapine oral disintegrating tablet (ODT), and this was increased to 20 mg a day—given as two equal divided doses a day. After 12 days of treatment on this medication as a primary antipsychotic, he began to make progress and became more compliant with medication and less aggressive and paranoid. Bob also showed better boundaries with peers and was able to participate in milieu therapy without being disruptive. He was eventually discharged to a community mental health center for follow-up—with wraparound services such as in-home therapy, substance use counseling groups and close medication management follow-up.

Considerations with the Use of Second-Generation Antipsychotics

Quetiapine [30]—with its shorter half-life, potential to provide a therapeutic sedation, and ability to be titrated rapidly—can be helpful in maintaining safety with relatively lower risk of inducing dystonia or extrapyramidal side effects, especially in a patient who is compliant with taking medication orally. The risks of prolonged QTc interval with rapid dose increases and concomitant agitation may increase the risk of a ventricular tachyarrhythmia, and EKG monitoring at baseline and therapeutic doses is indicated. Risperidone and Olanzapine [31, 32] may be used for more aggressive patients when the risk of assaultive behavior and aggression is high, with both medications being available in orally disintegrating tablet forms and the latter being additionally available in intramuscular form as well. Risperidone (half-life of 3 h, active metabolite 18 h) and Olanzapine (half-life of 30 h) also lend themselves to once-a-day dosing though twice a day dosing is often used by the child psychiatrist to minimize peak plasma levels and reduce the risk of dystonic reactions. Aripiprazole [33] has a more delayed onset of action and the oral form is not often preferred to manage acute aggression, and due to limited information and supply, intramuscular dosing has not been studied. Aripiprazole may nevertheless be of significant clinical importance due to its availability as a long-acting monthly injectable which is both safe and well tolerated in adolescents. This option might be practical, as well as acceptable to patients closer to the time of discharge once the acute stabilization is achieved. While we have limited data on the efficacy of Asenapine [34], it could be beneficial due to its oral disintegrating tablet form and sedative effect in a patient who might be agitated.

The maxim of "start low and go slow" is often not a luxury the child and adolescent psychiatrist can afford in these situations. Adjunctive medication to reduce aggression include Benzodiazepines, and Lorazepam is often used in the inpatient setting at doses of 2–8 mg/day to manage the acutely agitated or violent patient.

This psychiatrist often must consider that regular and concomitant use of tobacco products induces Cytochrome P450 1A2 (CYP1A2), which results in increased metabolism and lower levels of medications such as Clozapine, Olanzapine, and Haloperidol.

In contrast to the psychotimimetic and psychotogenic effects of THC, there is evidence that the use of cannabidiol might have a role in the prevention and delay of first episode psychosis due to its effects of enhancing the levels of endocannabinoid anandamide and desensitization of cannabinoid receptors, and antagonism at CB1 receptors. Leweke et al. found that the ability of cannabidiol to inhibit FAAH (fatty amino amide hydrolase) was as effective as Amisulpiride in the treatment of acute psychosis (both positive and negative symptoms) while having a favorable side effect profile—suggesting it might be a worthwhile alternative for the treatment of youth [35].

Management of Mood Disorders Associated with Cannabis Use

When co-occurring with cannabis use, mood disorders can be persistent and lead to avoidance of treatment. Young patients often expect that the psychiatrist will align with their parents and be quick to impose sanctions against their use of cannabis, which would be tied to limits set around their peers who share their habit and whom they regard as supports. In this regard, it is very helpful to lead with a clear explanation about the confidentiality around their disclosures around substance use and maintaining an open and curious position. Youth using substances often experience a breakdown in family support, including running away from home and thereby exposing themselves to the risk of trauma. The temperamental trait of avoidance and "seeking relief or escape" is frequently associated with both suicidal and substance use behavior. Another temperamental trait associated with suicide is impulsivity, which in conjunction with cognitive, affective, and behavioral traits of the teenager due to a relative deficit in cortical inhibitory processes results in a stronger libidinal drive, sensation seeking behavior, and aggression to self and others.

Antidepressants are often useful to the extent that patients are compliant with taking medication, and an explanation of how the medication needs to be taken consistently for it to be effective is important. The first line of treatment is usually a selective serotonin reuptake inhibitor such as Fluoxetine, Sertraline, or Escitalopram [36–38]. These medications are well tolerated and have a wide safety margin, though young patients have to be advised about the need for compliance and the delay in onset of the effects for 4–6 weeks. Youth often expect that the medication will improve mood and anxiety symptoms in a few days, and due to their need to see immediate results stemming from a developmentally driven impulsivity, may be prone to "give up" these medications prematurely.

Youth often use "vape" products containing cannabis concentrates and nicotine products interchangeably. Frequent association of nicotine use and Attention Deficit/Hyperactivity Disorder suggests that Bupropion/Bupropion XL may also have a role in the treatment of cannabis use disorders at doses of 100 to 400 mg/day, especially if associated with the use of nicotine.

Sleep disorders that emerge in the context of depression could benefit from the addition of Trazodone in smaller doses of 25 to 100 mg as an adjunct to manage insomnia. Mirtazapine has also been effective in teens who have struggles with the initiation or maintenance of sleep without cannabis or other soporifics in small samples. Other medications that involve norepinephrine transmission (Atomoxetine, Nefazodone) or combined norepinephrine/serotonin transmission (Venlafaxine) have been studied in adults and young adults, but these proved to be poorly tolerated and of limited efficacy.

The management of a Bipolar Mood disorder associated with the use of cannabis is often more complicated—with the emphasis on reducing high risk and self-endangering behavior. Substance use is often a critical predictor of outcomes in adolescent-onset Bipolar Disorder, and youth with Bipolar Disorder are more likely to use substances than those with unipolar depression. Due to the frequency of aggression, agitation, and sleep disturbances, atypical antipsychotics are often the first line of treatment. The considerations for their use are very similar to those described in the preceding section on the management of psychosis, as outlined previously in this chapter. Geller et al. studied the use of Lithium in youth assessed to have Bipolar Disorder and subsequent Substance Dependency Disorders and it was an efficacious treatment for both disorders [39]. In this study, Alcohol and Cannabis dependence were the most frequent substances used by participants.

There have been open-label and double-blind placebo-controlled trials of N Acetylcysteine (NAC), which have suggested doses of NAC at 2400 mg/day were potentially helpful in improving long-term outcomes. An open-label, pilot clinical trial found significant reductions in self-reported marijuana use and craving—but not in biomarkers of use—among 24 adolescents after 4 weeks of NAC, 1200 mg twice daily. The same researchers (Gray et al. 2012) conducted an 8-week, double-blind randomized controlled trial of 116 adolescents using NAC at 1200 mg twice daily with contingency management and noted that this intervention did double the odds of abstinence but had no effect on self-reported craving or use [40–47].

Conclusion

As mentioned at the start of this chapter, adolescent cannabis use complicates the clinical management of pre-existing psychiatric disorders and adds complexity to considerations of differential diagnosis. There is growing evidence for the impact of cannabis use during adolescence on mood changes, suicidal ideation, and psychosis. Though cannabis use is often considered societally "benign," child and adolescent psychiatrists in states with increased access to cannabis may see increasing rates of children and teenagers admitted to inpatient psychiatric units for these concerns. It is important to engage these patients in evidence-based substance treatment prior to or soon after discharge from inpatient psychiatric units. Specific interventions are covered in Chap. 5. Even when induced by Cannabis - psychosis, depression or other psychiatric symptoms may benefit from medication mangement and are not reason to withhold treatment with more conventional agents. Synthetic cannabinoids are also important for this population; they are covered in more detail in our "Cannabis in the Child and Adolescent Medical and Consultation-Liaison Settings" (Chap. 7).

Highlights Box 6.1 Key Points for Patient Psychoeducation

Adolescent-onset cannabis use significantly increases the risk of psychosis; risk even greater in those with genetic vulnerability to schizophrenia:

- Cannabis psychosis risk is increased by the following factors: earlier age onset, > frequency of use, use of > potency THC, familial risk for schizophrenia.
- Cannabis-induced psychosis in use without genetic vulnerability may be more likely to remit with cannabis cessation and have a less chronic

persistent course compared to cannabis-induced psychosis in use in those with genetic/familial risk of schizophrenia.

- Persistent cannabis use after initial onset of psychosis (regardless of schizophrenia risk) is less likely to remit psychosis and evolve into chronic psychotic illness.

Highlights Box 6.2 Key Points in Treatment and Management

The involvement of family and an extended network of support is often critical to the process of recovery in the case of Mood disorders or Psychosis complicated by substance abuse:

- It is critically important to make every effort to link and engage such patients in substance treatment post discharge and emphasize the importance of cessation to prognosis and illness severity.
- The treatment considerations in patients who present with an acute onset of psychosis do not differ very much from the management of those with a chronic prodrome—apart from the need for frequent or urgent use of medication to manage agitation and aggression.
- Atypical antipsychotics may be helpful for symptomatic management of cannabis-induced psychosis.
- Antidepressants can be helpful for the management of depressive symptoms related to (or preceding) cannabis use.
- NAC may be helpful for cannabis use and cravings.

References

1. Henquet C, Krabbendam L, Spauwen J, et al. Prospective cohort study of cannabis use, predisposition for psychosis, and psychotic symptoms in young people. BMJ. 2005;330(7481):11. https://doi.org/10.1136/bmj.38267.664086.63.
2. Wang GS, Davies SD, Halmo LS, Sass A, Mistry RD. Impact of marijuana legalization in Colorado on adolescent emergency and urgent care visits. J Adolesc Health. 2018;63(2):239–41. https://doi.org/10.1016/j.jadohealth.2017.12.010.
3. Wainberg M, Jacobs GR, di Forti M, Tripathy SJ. Cannabis, schizophrenia genetic risk, and psychotic experiences: a cross-sectional study of 109,308 participants from the UK biobank. Transl. Psychiatry. 2021;11(1):211. https://doi.org/10.1038/s41398-021-01330-w.
4. Starzer MSK, Nordentoft M, Hjorthøj C. Rates and predictors of conversion to schizophrenia or bipolar disorder following substance-induced psychosis. Am J Psychiatry. 2018;175(4):343–50. https://doi.org/10.1176/appi.ajp.2017.17020223.
5. Levine A, Clemenza K, Rynn M, Lieberman J. Evidence for the risks and consequences of adolescent cannabis exposure. J Am Acad Child Adolesc Psychiatry. 2017;56(3):214–25. https://doi.org/10.1016/j.jaac.2016.12.014.
6. Bagot KS, Milin R, Kaminer Y. Adolescent initiation of cannabis use and early-onset psychosis. Subst Abus. 2015;36(4):524–33. https://doi.org/10.1080/08897077.2014.995332.

7. Fergusson DM, Horwood LJ, Ridder EM. Tests of causal linkages between cannabis use and psychotic symptoms. Addiction. 2005;100(3):354–66. https://doi.org/10.1111/j.1360-0443.2005.01001.x.
8. Fergusson DM, Lynskey MT, Horwood LJ. The short-term consequences of early onset cannabis use. J Abnorm Child Psychol. 1996;24(4):499–512. https://doi.org/10.1007/BF01441571.
9. Andréasson S, Allebeck P, Engström A, Rydberg U. Cannabis and schizophrenia. A longitudinal study of Swedish conscripts. Lancet. 1987;2(8574):1483–6. https://doi.org/10.1016/s0140-6736(87)92620-1. PMID: 2892048
10. Arseneault L, Cannon M, Poulton R, Murray R, Caspi A, Moffitt TE. Cannabis use in adolescence and risk for adult psychosis: longitudinal prospective study. BMJ. 2002;325(7374):1212–3. https://doi.org/10.1136/bmj.325.7374.1212.
11. Di Forti M, Morgan C, Dazzan P, et al. High-potency cannabis and the risk of psychosis. Br J Psychiatry. 2009;195(6):488–91. https://doi.org/10.1192/bjp.bp.109.064220.
12. Di Forti M, Quattrone D, Freeman TP, et al. The contribution of cannabis use to variation in the incidence of psychotic disorder across Europe (EU-GEI): a multicentre case-control study. Lancet Psychiatry. 2019;6(5):427–36. https://doi.org/10.1016/S2215-0366(19)30048-3.
13. Gage SH, Hickman M, Zammit S. Association between cannabis and psychosis: epidemiologic evidence. Biol Psychiatry. 2016;79(7):549–56. https://doi.org/10.1016/j.biopsych.2015.08.001.
14. Moore TH, Zammit S, Lingford-Hughes A, et al. Cannabis use and risk of psychotic or affective mental health outcomes: a systematic review. Lancet. 2007;370(9584):319–28. https://doi.org/10.1016/S0140-6736(07)61162-3.
15. Bechtold J, Hipwell A, Lewis DA, Loeber R, Pardini D. Concurrent and sustained cumulative effects of adolescent marijuana use on subclinical psychotic symptoms. Am J Psychiatry. 2016;173(8):781–9. https://doi.org/10.1176/appi.ajp.2016.15070878.
16. D'Souza DC, Abi-Saab WM, Madonick S, et al. Delta-9-tetrahydrocannabinol effects in schizophrenia: implications for cognition, psychosis, and addiction. Biol Psychiatry. 2005;57(6):594–608. https://doi.org/10.1016/j.biopsych.2004.12.006.
17. Esmaeelzadeh S, Moraros J, Thorpe L, Bird Y. Examining the association and directionality between mental health disorders and substance use among adolescents and young adults in the U.S. and Canada-a systematic review and meta-analysis. J Clin Med. 2018;7(12):543. https://doi.org/10.3390/jcm7120543.
18. Sadock BJ, Sadock VA, Ruiz P. Kaplan and Sadock's concise textbook of clinical psychiatry. 4th ed. Philadelphia, PA: Wolters Kluwer; 2016.
19. Khantzian EJ. The self-medication hypothesis of substance use disorders: a reconsideration and recent applications. Harv Rev Psychiatry. 1997;4:231–44. https://doi.org/10.3109/10673229709030550.
20. Hooshmand S, Willoughby T, Good M. Does the direction of effects in the association between depressive symptoms and health-risk behaviors differ by behavior? A longitudinal study across the high school years. J Adolesc Health. 2012;50(2):140–7. https://doi.org/10.1016/j.jadohealth.2011.05.016.
21. Schoeler T, Theobald D, Pingault JB, Farrington DP, Coid JW, Bhattacharyya S. Developmental sensitivity to cannabis use patterns and risk for major depressive disorder in mid-life: findings from 40 years of follow-up. Psychol Med. 2018;48(13):2169–76. https://doi.org/10.1017/S0033291717003658.
22. Silins E, Horwood LJ, Patton GC, et al. Young adult sequelae of adolescent cannabis use: an integrative analysis. Lancet Psychiatry. 2014;1(4):286–93. https://doi.org/10.1016/S2215-0366(14)70307-4.
23. Gobbi G, Atkin T, Zytynski T, Wang S, Askari S, Boruff J, Ware M, Marmorstein N, Cipriani A, Dendukuri N, Mayo N. Association of cannabis use in adolescence and risk of depression,

anxiety, and suicidality in young adulthood: a systematic review and meta-analysis. JAMA Psychiat. 2019;76(4):426–34. https://doi.org/10.1001/jamapsychiatry.2018.4500.
24. Carvalho AF, Stubbs B, Vancampfort D, et al. Cannabis use and suicide attempts among 86,254 adolescents aged 12-15 years from 21 low- and middle-income countries. Eur Psychiatry. 2019;56:8–13. https://doi.org/10.1016/j.eurpsy.2018.10.006.
25. Rasic D, Weerasinghe S, Asbridge M, Langille DB. Longitudinal associations of cannabis and illicit drug use with depression, suicidal ideation and suicidal attempts among Nova Scotia high school students. Drug Alcohol Depend. 2013;129(1–2):49–53. https://doi.org/10.1016/j.drugalcdep.2012.09.009.
26. Adalberto AC, Suárez-Colorado YP, Caballero-Domínguez CC. Association between the use of cannabis and elevated suicide risk in high school adolescents from Santa Marta, Colombia. Biomedica. 2020;40(3):569–77.
27. Lawn W, Freeman TP, Pope RA, et al. Acute and chronic effects of cannabinoids on effort-related decision-making and reward learning: an evaluation of the cannabis 'amotivational' hypotheses. Psychopharmacology. 2016;233(19–20):3537–52. https://doi.org/10.1007/s00213-016-4383-x.
28. van Hell HH, Jager G, Bossong MG, et al. Involvement of the endocannabinoid system in reward processing in the human brain. Psychopharmacology. 2012;219(4):981–90. https://doi.org/10.1007/s00213-011-2428-8.
29. Johnston LD, O'Malley PM, Bachman JG, Schulenberg JE. Monitoring the future national results on adolescent drug use: overview of key findings, 2011. Ann Arbor: Institute for Social Research, The University of Michigan; 2012.
30. Quetiapine (Systemic). In: Lexi-Drugs. Lexi-Comp, Inc. Updated 31 Aug 2021. Accessed 31 Aug 2021.
31. Risperidone (Systemic). In: Lexi-Drugs. Lexi-Comp, Inc. Updated. 31 Aug 2021. Accessed 31 Aug 2021.
32. Olanzapine (Systemic). In: Lexi-Drugs. Lexi-Comp, Inc. Updated 31 Aug 2021. Accessed 31 Aug 2021.
33. Aripiprazole (Systemic). In: Lexi-Drugs. Lexi-Comp, Inc. Updated 31 Aug 2021. Accessed 31 Aug 2021.
34. Asenapine (Systemic). In: Lexi-Drugs. Lexi-Comp, Inc. Updated 17 Aug 2021. Accessed 31 Aug 2021.
35. Leweke FM, Piomelli D, Pahlisch F, et al. Cannabidiol enhances anandamide signaling and alleviates psychotic symptoms of schizophrenia. Transl. Psychiatry. 2012;2(3):e94. https://doi.org/10.1038/tp.2012.15.
36. Fluoxetine (Systemic). In: Lexi-Drugs. Lexi-Comp, Inc. Updated 31 Aug 2021. Accessed 31 Aug 2021.
37. Sertraline (Systemic). In: Lexi-Drugs. Lexi-Comp, Inc. Updated 31 Aug 2021. Accessed 31 Aug 2021.
38. Escitalopram (Systemic). In: Lexi-Drugs. Lexi-Comp, Inc. Updated 31 Aug 2021. Accessed 31 Aug 2021.
39. Geller B, Cooper TB, Sun K, Zimerman B, Frazier J, Williams M, Heath J. Double-blind and placebo-controlled study of lithium for adolescent bipolar disorders with secondary substance dependency. J Am Acad Child Adolesc Psychiatry. 1998;37(2):171–8. https://doi.org/10.1097/00004583-199802000-00009.
40. Gray KM, Carpenter MJ, Baker NL, et al. A double-blind randomized controlled trial of N-acetylcysteine in cannabis-dependent adolescents. Am J Psychiatry. 2012;169(8):805–12.
41. Lorazepam (Systemic). In: Lexi-Drugs. Lexi-Comp, Inc. Updated 28 Aug 2021. Accessed 31 Aug 2021.
42. Bupropion (Systemic). In: Lexi-Drugs. Lexi-Comp, Inc. Updated 27 Aug 2021. Accessed 31 Aug 2021.

43. Bupropion XL (Systemic). In: Lexi-Drugs. Lexi-Comp, Inc. Updated 27 Aug 2021. Accessed 27 Aug 2021.
44. Mirtazapine (Systemic). In: Lexi-Drugs. Lexi-Comp, Inc. Updated 27 Aug 2021. Accessed 31 Aug 2021.
45. Atomoxetine (Systemic). In: Lexi-Drugs. Lexi-Comp, Inc. Updated 13 Aug 2021. Accessed 31 Aug 2021.
46. Nefazodone (Systemic). In: Lexi-Drugs. Lexi-Comp, Inc. Updated 17 Aug 2021. Accessed 31 Aug 2021.
47. Venlafaxine (Systemic). In: Lexi-Drugs. Lexi-Comp, Inc. Updated 27 Aug 2021. Accessed 31 Aug 2021.

Clinical Considerations for Cannabis in the Child and Adolescent Consultation-Liaison Setting

7

Beau Carubia and Anne Penner

Clinical Case

"J.T." is a 12-year-old male with a known history of ADHD who initially presented to a pediatric emergency room along with his mother with a chief complaint of altered mental status. History gathered by the admitting physician included a two-day, acute onset of confusion, intermittent, vague auditory and visual hallucinations, and reported much increased "irritability and mood swings." Physical exam was notable for the patient appearing lethargic, with observed slight ataxia, as well as noted tachycardia and mydriasis. Laboratory studies done included a normal complete blood count (CBC) and complete metabolic panel (CMP), negative acetaminophen and salicylate levels, and a urine toxicology screen positive for cannabinoids. The patient's mother reported she had caught the patient "smoking a joint with a friend" approximately 2–3 weeks prior. A lumbar puncture was completed and noted to be unremarkable. While being evaluated in the emergency room, J.T. was intermittently agitated and, on one occasion, aggressed towards his nurse requiring the use of physical restraints and PRN medication. J.T. was placed on an overnight electroencephalogram (EEG) and admitted to the inpatient pediatric service with a planned magnetic resonance imaging (MRI) study ordered for later in the morning. Neurology and Psychiatry Consults were placed by the inpatient pediatric provider. Subsequently, the EEG and MRI are both read as normal. Upon further history gathering, the patient's older sister, who lives in the home, reports that J.T. had been using his father's "vape pen" over the course of the past 1 to 2 weeks. J.T.'s father is contacted and reports the vape pen that

B. Carubia (✉) · A. Penner
Department of Psychiatry, Children's Hospital Colorado, University of Colorado School of Medicine, Aurora, CO, USA
e-mail: beau.carubia@childrenscolorado.org; anne.penner@cuanschutz.edu

P. Riggs, T. Thant (eds.), *Cannabis in Psychiatric Practice*, Psychiatry Update 3,
https://doi.org/10.1007/978-3-031-04874-6_7

was stolen was actually filled with cannabis cartridges that the father identifies as "dabs" or dab concentrates. The pediatric team is now asking for recommendations for management of AMS and agitation.

Introduction

Any time a pediatric patient presents to a medical setting with the chief complaint of an acute change in mental status or behavior, it is likely that a broad differential will set in motion the use of multiple laboratory and diagnostic imaging studies, and possibly even invasive procedures (i.e., a lumbar puncture). Why is this the case? Simply put, there tends to be a level of hidden pressure on pediatric providers to quickly determine the cause of the symptoms and not to miss any serious medical conditions. This clinical scenario in pediatric medical settings will be especially familiar to those who serve as psychiatric consultants to emergency rooms or inpatient pediatric services. Severe alterations in mental status, and concern about substance use, can be very distressing for patients, families, and pediatric medical providers. This chapter will highlight key clinical considerations for providers including cannabis use patterns in adolescents, review of the clinical presentation of acute intoxications, and discussion of management strategies in the medical setting. Some topics will be referenced in this chapter but explored in more depth in others, such as cannabis hyperemesis, management of cannabis-related agitation, and outpatient treatment of cannabis use disorders (please see Chaps. 5, 6, and 7).

J.T.'s case highlights the difficulty of triaging and assessing a pediatric patient presenting with acute changes in mentation and behavior. Initially, his positive urine drug screen was potentially explained by a known, previous use, and subsequent medical evaluations were pursued. As will be explained in the chapter to come, the rates of cannabis use, both intentional and unintentional, are dramatically increasing causing illness in the medical setting. These clinical presentations in the pediatric and adolescent populations point to the importance of pediatric providers being prepared with increased awareness and management strategies to best support youth presenting with similar concerns.

Product Types and Concentrations

It is important for psychiatrists practicing in the inpatient consultation-liaison setting to be familiar with different cannabis products and comfortable with asking about formulation concentrations as it can help guide assessment and treatments in pediatric populations (covered later in this chapter).

The use of a variety of different cannabis products, in addition to varying concentrations of these products, has become particularly concerning within the pediatric population. As described in earlier chapters, delta-9-tetrahydrocannabinol (THC) is the most psychoactive cannabinoid and Cannabis sativa is the most commonly used recreational strain of cannabis [1]. THC concentrations can vary widely within each product, but generally speaking, the typical THC content in a grown marijuana plant may range from 12% to 20%, in non-solvent produced concentrates from 39% to 60%, and in solvent (i.e., butane, propane) produced concentrates from 39% to 80% [1]. It is no longer adequate to ask pediatric patients simply if they use marijuana; rather, we must further explore in detail what product and what concentration of THC is being used. Dried marijuana leaves may be smoked out of a hollowed-out cigar [blunt] or rolled into cigarette paper [joint]. Hashish, which is a marijuana plant extract containing psychoactive resins, can be smoked, vaporized, or consumed via oral ingestion. Hash oil is a cannabis concentrate that is extracted from hashish, basically forming a concentrated resin extract which can be smoked, vaporized, ingested orally, or used via a transdermal route. Of increasing concern, numerous vaporizable cannabis concentrates have become more widely available and carry the common names of Dabs, Shatter, Wax, Butane Hash Oil, and numerous others. These concentrates are extracted from the plant and concentrated with volatile organic solvents, like propane and butane [2]. Dabs, for example, are waxy resins that can easily have THC concentrations >70% [3]. The vaporizable cannabis concentrates are commonly used with vape pens or as electronic (e-cig) cartridges [1]. Edibles are commonly seen as foods infused with cannabis extracts (i.e., brownies, candies, etc.) and these products can easily contain 10–20 times a typical THC dose [2]. There is no federal regulation of the packaging of these items and they are often made to mimic non-THC containing food items [2]. Lastly, the Synthetic Cannabinoid Receptor Agonists (SCRAs), commonly known as "synthetics" are growing in popularity among pediatric populations.

Synthetic Cannabinoid Receptor Agonists (SCRAs)

SCRAs are more commonly known by names of K2, Spice, Black Mamba, Kush, Kronic, as well as many others. These products are typically engineered from a plant-derived material that is then mixed with engineered substances similar to synthetic THC [1]. A paper published in 2019 reported as many as 180 different SCRA products have been identified [4]. The SCRAs are known to be full agonists to both CB-1 and CB-2 receptors, rendering them with much higher potencies compared to THC products, which are only partial agonists [2, 3]. Reports vary widely regarding potency of the SCRAs, with a range anywhere from 2–800 times the potency of THC [5]. Given the increased potency of these products, the potential for more acute toxicity presentations becomes increasingly likely. From 2010 to 2015, a multicenter, hospital-based registry of toxicology consultations reported the frequency of the following clinical symptoms in 277 identified cases with a known, single agent synthetic cannabinoid exposure: agitation, coma, toxic psychosis or other nervous system finding (seizures, hallucination) (66%), bradycardia, tachycardia, other cardiovascular finding (17%), rhabdomyolysis (6%), respiratory depression (5%), and acute kidney injury (4%) [6]. Given the increased use of these products in the pediatric population, providers must become acutely aware of the clinical signs of acute intoxications.

Pediatric Clinical Presentations

Acute Intoxications

Pediatric patients presenting to emergency room or inpatient medical settings with cannabis intoxication, whether intentional, recreational, or exploratory, may challenge providers initially in terms of clinical diagnosis given the incredibly broad differential to consider. Common signs of cannabis intoxication may include poor concentration, distorted perception, hyperemesis, euphoria, increased appetite, anxiety, paranoia, tachycardia, dry mouth, conjunctival injection, sedation, respiratory depression, cardiotoxicity, pain relief, and possibly psychotic symptoms [1, 7]. Other symptoms that have been described in case studies include ataxia, mydriasis, and hypotonia [8]. Onset of abrupt or acute psychotic symptoms has also been described with cannabis intoxication and may be linked to potency and amount of product used [9]. As is evident, some of these symptoms are nonspecific and may be seen in many organic presentations including other toxidromes, delirium, and encephalopathic disease processes. Hopefully this highlights the need for the clinical practice of maintaining a broad differential as clinical histories are gathered to best inform initial diagnostic explorations.

Unintentional/Exploratory Intoxications

Unintentional or exploratory intoxications of cannabis are far more common in very young children (typically in the age range of 0–12 years of age) and are reported as accidental ingestions. Most of the literature surrounding unintentional or "exploratory" ingestions focus on younger children, in the age range of 0–12 years with reviews of clinical presentations to emergency medical settings as well as reviews of cases reported to regional poison control (RPC) centers. In addition, a good deal of data at state levels is beginning to show the impact of decriminalization of marijuana use. In 2009, five years post decriminalization of marijuana, Colorado saw it's rate of cannabis exposure cases reported to RPC's increase by 34%. In addition, annual RPC pediatric marijuana exposure cases showed a greater than five-fold increase from 2009 to 2015 [10]. Wang et al. also found unintentional ingestions of recreational cannabis accounted for almost half of all cannabis toxicity cases admitted to Children's Hospital Colorado from 2014 to 2015—the year after Colorado passed legislation legalizing recreational cannabis use [10]. Adolescent urgent care and emergency room visits secondary to marijuana exposure increased from 1.8 to 4.9 per 1000 visits from 2009 to 2015 [10]. According to another author, exposure of cannabis products to children rose 148% nationwide from 2006 to 2013, and by 610% in states that allow medical cannabis [11]. As is evident, exploratory ingestions of cannabis products have also shown a dramatic increase over the past 15–20 years. Grigbsy et al. cite numerous authors reporting the following symptoms in unintentional ingestions: sedation and increased lethargy, ataxia, tachycardia, hyperemesis, as well as rare CNS depression, and respiratory depression (at times requiring intubation) [7]. In 2017, a systematic review was conducted by Richards et al. to summarize the clinical presentations of unintentional cannabis ingestions in children (including 3582 youth, aged 12 years or younger) [12]. The authors found lethargy as the most common presenting symptom (71%), followed by ataxia (14%), and identified tachycardia, mydriasis, hypotonia, and hypoventilation as other, possible presenting symptoms [12]. In any medical environment including emergency room and inpatient settings, cannabis toxicity should be included on the differential diagnosis with the sudden onset of any of these clinical symptoms.

Initial Evaluation for Intoxication

When a child presents to the emergency room or is admitted to the medical floor with symptoms of cannabis intoxication, the diagnosis may not be clear. At the very start of a medical encounter obtaining a thorough history, physical, and basic laboratory data is necessary. Consultation with a child and adolescent psychiatrist with expertise in medical and psychiatric presentations may be necessary to evaluate for possible etiologies (Table 7.1). A history should include a thorough history of present illness including a careful timeline of symptoms, presence of cannabis products in the home (especially edibles), route of cannabis ingestion if known, and any co-ingestions. Some helpful questions to ask in the history include how the individual obtained the substance, who they were with, do they use other substances, and/or if there is a possibility this episode of substance use could have included another substance causing another toxidrome (Table 7.2).

Additionally, in the evaluation of a child or adolescent, it is important to know as much about the environment and surrounding circumstances as possible. What is the developmental level of the child? Who lives with the child? Who has custody and medical decision-making for the child? In an older child or adolescent, what was the intention behind the ingestion? This will help determine what safety precautions are required while the rest of the management plan takes place.

Laboratory Studies

Diagnosis of a cannabis ingestion or exposure is primarily a clinical diagnosis. With a history of sudden alteration in mental status with associated symptoms consistent

Table 7.1 Other common reasons for child and adolescent CL consultation related to cannabis

- Initial onset psychosis
- Chronic/severe cannabis use disorder or substance use disorder with associated suicidality, behavioral issues, or other psychiatric symptoms (mood changes, anxiety)
- Altered mental status or delirium
- Recurrent hyperemesis
- Pulmonary complications: EVALI, asthma exacerbation/hemoptysis

Table 7.2 Highlights for care of pediatric patients with cannabis exposures

- Obtain a very detailed history of presenting illness including detailed substance abuse history (of both patients and parents)
- Labs: Consider: CMP, CBC, TSH, EKG, urine and serum toxicology panels
- Treatment recommendations
  - Mild-moderate: Mostly supportive cares and environmental control measures
  - More severe: Consider medication management: Benzodiazepines
- Treatment recommendations following the acute medical management of patients meeting criteria for cannabis use disorder (CUD):
  - warm handoff to co-occurring treatment utilizing motivational interviewing
  - Post-discharge treatment with motivational enhancement treatment, cognitive-behavioral therapy, and contingency management (please see Chap. 5)

with cannabis intoxication, early evaluation likely will include: basic labs, electrocardiogram, and serum and urine toxicology screening. Early urine drug screen may be helpful. In young children with no substance use history, this may be diagnostic, and save a child from more invasive neurologic studies. However, the confirmatory test in this population would be a gas chromatography-mass spectrometry test for THC specifically. This may be delayed in some clinical settings [10]. Additionally, in older children and adolescents, who may use cannabis on a regular or semi-regular basis, this may be less immediately helpful since THC metabolites can be detected for on average 12.9 days for light users and 31.5 days for heavy users (Table 7.2) [13].

Given the limitations of immediate lab testing, it is even more important to make the diagnosis clinically with a vigilance for other causes of altered mental status. Reasons to complete a lumbar puncture, head imaging, and further neurological consultation include atypical history, focal neurological exam findings, abnormal movements, seizures, fever, deteriorating or persistently altered mental status. Psychiatry consultation services, regional poison control centers, and medical toxicologists all play an important role and should be involved in the assessment and planning for ongoing workup and management.

Clinical Management

Acute Intoxication

Approach

The management of young children with suspected cannabis intoxication due to unintended or accidental exposure/ingestion is primarily determined by severity of symptoms and a judgment of the person's current clinical stability. Supportive care is the cornerstone of treatment, with attention to the individual's symptoms. When approaching a child with any ingestion, or a suspected cannabis ingestion, a history including the entire context of the child's presentation is necessary. This can include obtaining details around the amount and type (formulation) of cannabis ingested to better understand the timeframe of clinical symptoms. A young child is more likely to be an unintentional ingestion while an adolescent patient may have misjudged the amount of cannabis they ingested.

There are additional clinical management factors in the pediatric population as it relates to inadvertent or unintended cannabis exposure/ingestion in young children. For example, should an episode of cannabis ingestion be reported to authorities? There is a lack of consensus among pediatric health care professionals and in state legal standards on the role of reporting unintentional ingestions to child protective agencies, especially in areas where the substance is legalized or decriminalized for the caregivers [10, 14]. However, there is always space for clinician judgment to consider if there is evidence of neglect in the case of an ingestion. This underscores the importance of understanding the child's environment and context to know if there is any reportable signs of abuse, neglect, or unsafe behavior going on in the home that could fall within one's jurisdiction for reporting standards [15].

Management

For mild to moderate ingestions with relatively mild symptoms, most patients (both children and adolescents) can be treated with supportive care. This is primarily done by reducing stimulation and offering reassurance and reorientation. If the child is admitted to the medical floor, then this is often accomplished by employing a dedicated staff person to monitor the patient and provide redirection and verbal prompts, lowering the lights, decreasing sounds, and limiting unnecessary exams or questions. For more moderate to severe ingestions, characterized by frank paranoia, tachycardia, agitation that becomes unsafe, then pharmacological management is recommended. Benzodiazepines are the first-line management for hospitalized patients with severe intoxication (Table 7.2) [16].

In addition to observing and monitoring the severity of the symptoms, the age of the child can be a factor in the course of the ingestion. A very young child may present with respiratory suppression, and even coma. They should be immediately referred to the pediatric intensive care unit and specialists. A consultation with a medical toxicologist is also useful for severe cannabis intoxication, or even intensive care physicians if there is concern for respiratory compromise in very young patients.

There is overall very mixed evidence for the appropriate next steps in psychiatric management for children and adolescents in a medical setting [17]. The use of screening and brief interventions is of particular interest to medical systems given the short though frequent encounters in a medical system allowing for a population health approach to addressing pediatric patients using substances. In a prospective, randomized and controlled trial by Berstein et al., a 20-min intervention based in Motivational Interviewing (MI) principles with a peer educator in a pediatric ER, found promising results in reducing marijuana consumption on follow-up [18]. However, a meta-analysis including the Bernstein paper did not find MI to be effective as a brief intervention in the medical setting for reducing cannabis consumption days [19]. These mixed results leave us with unclear evidence guidance when it comes to effective interventions for cannabis through brief psychotherapeutic interventions in the medical setting.

Pharmacological management of cannabis use disorder is similarly challenged in the pediatric population with limitations in high quality evidence. There are no FDA approved medications for cannabis use disorder in children or adolescents, despite its prevalence amongst youth and adults. The two most studied medication strategies in a pediatric population are *N*-acetylcysteine (NAC) and Gabapentin [20]. In a psychiatric consultation, it may be reasonable to assess if a patient is interested in medication management geared towards reducing cravings or the acute effects of withdrawal. Use of medications such as dronabinol for cannabis withdrawal management has not been well studied in pediatrics, so it is not recommended at this time.

Conclusion

Studies support increased pediatric exposures (particularly with cannabis edibles) in states following legalization despite increased regulations and improved child-resistant packaging regulations [10, 21]. As more states pass laws to legalize or decriminalize marijuana, it is clear that additional safeguards for children will be needed to prevent harm from unintentional exposures, or the mental health considerations discussed in other chapters of this book. An additional unique consideration in the pediatric medical setting is how legalization of medical and recreational marijuana for adults affects children. As highlighted in our clinical case above, it is important for psychiatrists in pediatric consultation-liaison settings to develop competency and comfort with assessing cannabis use (including formulations, routes of use, and concentrations), severity of use (as evidenced by medical sequelae such as altered mental status, EVALI, and hyperemesis syndrome), and initial strategies for managing cannabis use disorder.

Highlights Box 7.1 Key Points for Patient Psychoeducation

- There is increased pediatric cannabis-related exposures following legalization and decriminalization of cannabis.
- Unintentional or exploratory intoxications of cannabis are far more common in very young children (typically in the age range of 0–12 years of age).
- Edibles are of particular concern in pediatric exposures. Edibles are commonly seen as foods infused with cannabis extracts (i.e., brownies, candies, etc.) and these products can easily contain 10–20 times a typical THC dose.
- There is a lack of consensus among pediatric health care professionals and in state legal standards on the role of reporting unintentional ingestions to child protective agencies, especially in areas where the substance is legalized or decriminalized for the caregivers.

Highlights Box 7.2 Key Points in Treatment and Management

- Lethargy is the most common presenting symptom of unintentional pediatric cannabis exposures followed by ataxia.
- In any medical environment including emergency room and inpatient settings, cannabis toxicity should be included on the differential diagnosis with the sudden onset of lethargy, ataxia, tachycardia, hyperemesis, mydriasis, hypotonia, hypoventilation, and more rarely CNS depression.
- In cases of possible cannabis exposure, clinicians should obtain a very detailed history of presenting illness including detailed substance use history of both patient and parents.
- Possible labs to consider include: CMP, CBC, TSH, EKG, Urine and Serum toxicology panels.

References

1. Dharmapuri S, Miller K, Klein JD. Marijuana and the pediatric population. Pediatrics. 2020;146:2.
2. Blohm E, Sell P, Neavyn M. Cannabinoid toxicity in pediatrics. Curr Opin Pediatr. 2019;31(2):256–61.
3. Wong KU, Baum CR. Acute cannabis toxicity. Pediatr Emerg Care. 2019;35(11):799–804.
4. Potts A, Cano C, Thomas S, Hill S. Synthetic cannabinoid receptor agonists: classification and nomenclature. Clin Toxicol. 2020;58(2):82–98.
5. Musselman ME, Hampton JP. "Not for human consumption": a review of emerging designer drugs. Pharmacotherapy. 2014;34(7):745–57.
6. Riederer AM, Campleman SL, Carlson RG, Boyer EW, Manini AF, Wax PM, et al. Acute poisonings from synthetic cannabinoids—50 US Toxicology Investigators Consortium registry sites, 2010–2015. MMWR Morb Mortal Wkly Rep. 2016;65(27):692.
7. Grigsby TM, Hoffmann LM, Moss MJ. Marijuana use and potential implications of marijuana legalization. Pediatr Rev. 2020;41(2):61–72.
8. Foster BC, Abramovici H, Harris CS. Cannabis and cannabinoids: kinetics and interactions. Am J Med. 2019;132(11):1266–70.
9. D'Souza DC, Perry E, MacDougall L, Ammerman Y, Cooper T, Braley G, et al. The psychotomimetic effects of intravenous delta-9-tetrahydrocannabinol in healthy individuals: implications for psychosis. Neuropsychopharmacology. 2004;29(8):1558–72.
10. Wang GS, Le Lait MC, Deakyne SJ, Bronstein AC, Bajaj L, Roosevelt G. Unintentional pediatric exposures to marijuana in Colorado, 2009-2015. JAMA Pediatr. 2016;170(9):e160971.
11. Onders B, Casavant MJ, Spiller HA, Chounthirath T, Smith GA. Marijuana exposure among children younger than six years in the United States. Clin Pediatr. 2016;55(5):428–36.
12. Richards JR, Smith NE, Moulin AK. Unintentional cannabis ingestion in children: a systematic review. J Pediatr. 2017;190:142–52.
13. Grotenhermen F. Pharmacokinetics and pharmacodynamics of cannabinoids. Clin Pharmacokinet. 2003;42(4):327–60.
14. Wood JN, Pecker LH, Russo ME, Henretig F, Christian CW. Evaluation and referral for child maltreatment in pediatric poisoning victims. Child Abuse Negl. 2012;36(4):362–9.
15. Pélissier F, Claudet I, Pélissier-Alicot A-L, Franchitto N. Parental cannabis abuse and accidental intoxications in children: prevention by detecting neglectful situations and at-risk families. Pediatr Emerg Care. 2014;30(12):862–6.

16. Wang GS, Post T. Cannabis (marijuana): acute intoxication. UpToDate [online]. 2019.
17. Stockings E, Hall WD, Lynskey M, Morley KI, Reavley N, Strang J, et al. Prevention, early intervention, harm reduction, and treatment of substance use in young people. Lancet Psychiatry. 2016;3(3):280–96.
18. Bernstein E, Edwards E, Dorfman D, Heeren T, Bliss C, Bernstein J. Screening and brief intervention to reduce marijuana use among youth and young adults in a pediatric emergency department. Acad Emerg Med. 2009;16(11):1174–85.
19. Gayes LA, Steele RG. A meta-analysis of motivational interviewing interventions for pediatric health behavior change. J Consult Clin Psychol. 2014;82(3):521.
20. Gray KM, Watson NL, Carpenter MJ, LaRowe SD. N-acetylcysteine (NAC) in young marijuana users: an open-label pilot study. Am J Addict. 2010;19(2):187.
21. Wang GS, Hoyte C, Roosevelt G, Heard K. The continued impact of marijuana legalization on unintentional pediatric exposures in Colorado. Clin Pediatr (Phila). 2019;58(1):114–6.

Part III

Cannabis in Adult Mental Health Settings: Outpatient Mental Health Setting

Disease Course and Prognosis

8

Matthew Shirazi and David Riedford

Clinical Case

"B" is a 26-year-old man with a history of both anxiety and depression symptoms since around age 18, developing concurrently with graduation from high school and a lack of concrete plans for the future. At that time, B sought psychiatric medication treatments initially from his PCP, who noted symptoms of generalized anxiety disorder (GAD), more so than depressive symptoms. After two partial and somewhat ineffective SSRI trials, B visited a general psychiatrist who confirmed the GAD diagnosis and attempted treatment with an SNRI, later augmentation with buspirone, and a referral to cognitive behavioral therapy. B had smoked cannabis flower in late high school although he did not use it consistently, but upon becoming more disillusioned with his consistent anxiety symptoms, he considered this as a possible alternative treatment. Visiting his local dispensary, he initially tried higher-potency cannabis flower, thinking it was helpful intermittently. He later tried vaporized concentrates with a higher THC percentage, hoping this would in turn relieve his anxiety for longer periods. B was later unsure if his anxiety was episodically worse between uses of the concentrate, which led him back to his previous psychiatrist to discuss the interactions of cannabis with his anxiety disorder.

M. Shirazi (✉)
Department of Psychiatry, UCHealth Medical Center of the Rockies, University of Colorado School of Medicine, Fort Collins, CO, USA
e-mail: matthew.shirazi@cuanschutz.edu

D. Riedford
Department of Psychiatry, University of Colorado School of Medicine, Aurora, CO, USA
e-mail: David.Riedford@cuanschutz.edu

P. Riggs, T. Thant (eds.), *Cannabis in Psychiatric Practice*, Psychiatry Update 3,
https://doi.org/10.1007/978-3-031-04874-6_8

Significance to Current Clinical Practice

As policies in the United States shift with regard to legalization of marijuana and other cannabis products, it has become increasingly more relevant to address how the use of cannabinoid substances may impact individuals who currently have or may be at risk for developing a psychiatric disorder. The most recent comprehensive report on the impacts of cannabis use in psychiatric illness was published by the National Academies of Sciences, Engineering, and Medicine in 2017. This report looked at previously published data on schizophrenia and other psychotic disorders, bipolar and related disorders, depressive disorders, anxiety disorders, and posttraumatic stress disorder (PTSD), and how cannabis use may worsen, or determine the course of, each illness. Studies were compiled summarizing current data for both risk of new onset of each of these illnesses in relation to cannabis use, and the impact on severity of disease course with cannabis use [1]. In the following section, we will summarize the findings of this report, highlighting key studies included in the report, and we will also include more recent findings that were not available at the time of that report.

Psychotic Disorders

Of the psychiatric illnesses that have been studied in association with cannabis use, the most heavily researched have been schizophrenia spectrum disorders. The 2017 report entitled "The Health Effects of Cannabis and Cannabinoids" compiled data from five systematic reviews, two cohort studies, and a case-control study, and found consistently across these studies that there was a high statistical association between cannabis users and the onset of schizophrenia or other psychotic disorders, noting a particularly increased risk for individuals who used more frequently [1]. A notable study included in this analysis was that of Di Forti et al., a case-control trial of 410 patients, which found that patients with first-episode psychosis were more likely to have used cannabis, more likely to be daily users, and more likely to be users of high-potency cannabinoids [2]. A more recent study by Di Forti et al. had comparable findings and included data from multiple sites across Europe [3]. While cannabis use can itself induce more transient psychotic symptoms, current literature suggests that cannabis-induced psychosis can later progress to presentations akin to schizophrenia in 41.2% of cases [4].

Previous literature exploring the impacts of cannabis use on the disease course of schizophrenia spectrum disorders has separated the impacts into three subcategories: positive symptoms, negative symptoms, and cognition. Research on the effects of cannabis use on positive symptoms has been somewhat mixed, with some studies demonstrating a slight association between cannabis use and increased severity of positive symptoms, while others did not demonstrate any statistically significant association [1]. There are fewer studies on the impacts of negative symptoms as compared to positive symptoms, but there is no indication from current published literature that cannabis use has a significant impact on the severity of negative symptoms [1]. Interestingly, when examining the impacts of cannabis use on cognition in schizophrenia and related disorders, a systematic review found that some areas of cognitive performance were actually improved with cannabis use [1, 5].

Bipolar and Related Disorders

The risk of onset of bipolar disorder with cannabis use is less clear. In a systematic review of two studies, Gibbs et al. found that the risk of new onset manic symptoms was nearly three times higher for cannabis users than non-cannabis users in individuals with no history of bipolar disorder. However, these findings were described as tentative by the authors due to the limited data available [6]. A retrospective cohort study utilizing data from the National Epidemiologic Survey on Alcohol and Related Conditions (NESARC) demonstrated that cannabis use within the past year was associated with higher risk of onset of bipolar disorder, but the risk was no longer statistically significant when adjusting for sociodemographic and clinic variables [7]. As a result, the authors of the 2017 report on the impacts of cannabis use in psychiatric disease concluded there was only limited evidence for an association between cannabis use and the onset of bipolar disorder [1]. However, there have been multiple studies linking cannabis use to an earlier age of onset of bipolar disorder, as highlighted by a systematic review from 2019 of 53 studies on bipolar disorder [8].

Compared to risk of onset of bipolar disorder, there is better evidence for an association between cannabis use and worsening disease course in bipolar disorder. Gibbs et al. in a systematic review of three studies found that cannabis use was associated with increased likelihood of mania (nearly three times as likely, OR 2.97), increased severity of manic episodes, and increased duration of manic episodes [6]. A 2015 longitudinal study of 1922 patients indicated that recovery and remission rates were lower among current users and recurrence rates were higher; it also found time to remission was increased [9]. Cannabis use disorder has also been associated with an increased number of depressive and manic or hypomanic episodes over 1 year [10].

Depressive Disorders

Depressive disorders are quite common, and therefore the impacts of cannabis use on disease onset and disease course are highly relevant. The current 12-month prevalence for major depressive disorder alone in the United States is 10.4%, with a lifetime prevalence of 20.6% [11]. Current literature suggests an increased risk of onset of a depressive disorder with cannabis use, as well as increased risk for suicidal ideation and suicide attempts (see Chap. 10 for more information on cannabis use and suicide risk) [1]. A systematic review by Lev-Ran et al. looked at 14 prospective longitudinal studies and, in a pooled odds ratio of ten of these studies, found a small but statistically significant increase in risk (OR = 1.17) for developing a depressive disorder among cannabis users. They also found that in a pooled odds ratio of seven of these studies, heavy cannabis use was associated with an even greater risk (OR = 1.62) of onset of depressive disorder [12]. However, data for risk of worsening disease course in depressive disorders is more limited. A longitudinal study published in 2017 using NESARC data found that in individuals with major depressive disorder, cannabis users did not have substantially different outcomes in terms of remission (as compared to nonusers), but the level of cannabis use was associated with an increased number of depressive symptoms at follow-up, particularly certain symptoms (including anhedonia, changes in weight, sleep difficulties, and psychomotor problems). Additionally, cannabis users had an earlier age of onset of major depressive disorder (compared to nonusers), which was younger still for individuals with cannabis use disorder. However, the number of lifetime episodes of major depression did not differ significantly among the groups [13].

Anxiety Disorders

Anxiety disorders are another major area of interest, with an estimated lifetime prevalence of 31.6% of any anxiety disorder in the United States, although this data was based on DSM-IV-TR criteria, which included diagnoses of OCD and PTSD (lifetime prevalence of 2.3% and 5.7%, respectively) [14]. The 2017 report by the National Academies of Sciences, Engineering, and Medicine concluded that there was some evidence to suggest that cannabis use does increase the risk of developing an anxiety disorder (based on a systematic review of 5 longitudinal studies), but the strongest evidence was for development of social anxiety disorder (which was a finding in three separate primary studies) [1]. The effect of cannabis use on disease course in anxiety disorders is less clear. The 2017 report by the National Academies of Sciences, Engineering, and Medicine cited one prospective study of college students which found no association between cannabis use and anxiety symptoms [1]. A retrospective study from 2017 (which was not included in that report) found that decreasing cannabis use among individuals with cannabis use disorder led to improvement in anxiety symptoms, but did not lead to significant improvements in quality of life [15]. The above case of "B" is a good example of how individuals with anxiety disorders may turn to cannabis for symptomatic relief, with current data suggesting that having an anxiety disorder increases both the risk of cannabis use (OR = 1.24) and the development of a cannabis use disorder (OR = 1.68). This same study also found that cannabis users were more likely to report anxiety at follow-up, which could be a possible explanation for "B's" cycle of escalating use, exhibited by both his increased frequency of use and increased concentration of substances used, all the while reporting persistent symptoms of anxiety [16].

Trauma- and Stressor-Related Disorders

The current data on the effects of cannabis use on PTSD is fairly limited. One prospective study has linked cannabis use with increased incidence of developing PTSD, and there is some limited evidence which associates cannabis use with worsened symptoms in those who have a previous diagnosis of PTSD [17]. A large observational cohort study by Wilkinson et al. of 2276 veterans found that 4 months after discharge from an intensive PTSD program, individuals who started using or continued to use cannabis had significantly worse symptoms of PTSD than those who had stopped using or had never used. Those who started using cannabis after discharge also exhibited violent behavior more frequently [18].

ADHD and Cannabis

Increasingly, ADHD and attentional disorders are being recognized, diagnosed, and treated in the adult psychiatric population—many providers also note a concurrence of these disorders with substance use [19]. The presence of an ADHD diagnosis is generally thought to complicate the treatment of substance use, and there is also data to suggest that use of cannabis and other substances may render ADHD treatment less effective [19]. Smaller studies have specifically investigated a connection between ADHD and presentation for cannabis use treatment, such as the estimation of prevalence performed by Notzon and colleagues in 2020. This study found an increased prevalence for ADHD of 34–46% in those presenting for cannabis treatment compared to a prevalence for ADHD of 2.5–5.0% in the general population [20]. Clearly, clinical management for this comorbidity must be considered, as is addressed elsewhere in this text.

Cannabinoids as Treatment

As this topic is covered extensively in another chapter, we will only briefly summarize findings from our literature search. Current literature suggests some benefit of CBD on symptoms of anxiety [21], as well as improvement in nightmares associated with PTSD [17]. However, CBD showed no benefit in psychotic illnesses, and it worsened symptoms of depression [21]. This is clearly a field of research which will require further data and time.

Treatment Approach and Patient Psychoeducation

As clinicians may have already experienced, discussing pitfalls of cannabis use with patients can be difficult. Those currently using cannabis may feel it is helpful or at least not deleterious, and they may have suspicions about prescribing providers attempting to "push" prescription medications over other treatments. With an increasing number of channels for obtaining information regarding cannabis, one role of psychiatric care may be to counsel patients on longitudinal outcomes of use. This requires a balanced approach, and it may be best undertaken by asking patients what they hope to gain from use. In the cases of those seeking relief from anxiety or depression symptoms most especially, citing the rich body of research in this chapter may be a fruitful approach. Conversely, harm reduction or "rolling with resistance" with those who choose to continue to use cannabis more recreationally may also be of value. Lastly, we as counselors of patients need to explore where our limited time and resources for psychoeducation may best be spent.

It is also important to consider why our patients would have begun to use cannabis at all—these reasons can be quite varied in nature. Of course, some people may use any substance recreationally, and they may have differing opinions about negative consequences, if any. For others, especially the patients most addressed in this chapter, use may represent a means to try to reduce suffering. Friends, relatives, or others may have suggested a "medical marijuana" approach, and patients may well now find themselves seeking other opinions or advice. Understanding and aligning with why patients use any substance, without undue judgement, is generally a more impactful approach when patients want to cut back or cease use.

In such instances, how best to approach the patient may depend on the provider and the patient, as well as their relation in a dyad. One can imagine working with adolescents, adults in a psychodynamic setting, or in a consultation role as being quite different. Approaches such as basic psychoeducation and appealing to physical health may be among the easiest entry points. Again, perhaps owing to cannabis industry efforts or societal normalization, cannabis is sometimes perceived as less physically harmful than tobacco or other smoked-plant material. Depending upon the relationship between the patient and provider, appealing to a personal wish for general wellness for the patient can also be of help. Below is a figure the author (M.S.) has sometimes drawn or referenced with patients, more so in a consultation model, to illustrate the data as a whole and the multifactorial impacts of cannabis use:

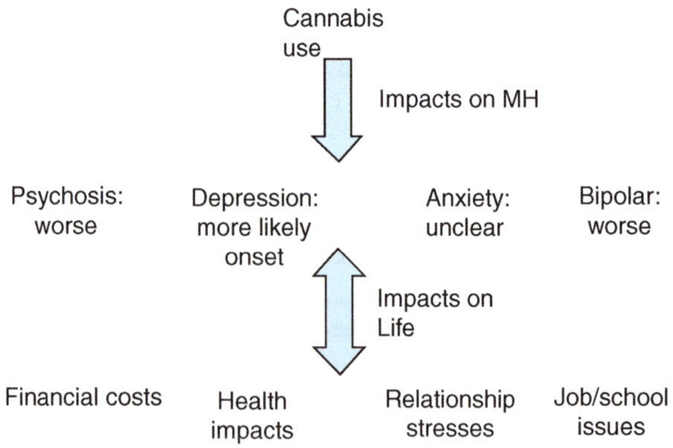

The above diagram can be drawn quickly with the patient in the room, with customization to highlight their particular diagnosis or largest area of life impact. Furthermore, details can be added, such as actual costs of use or known health impacts, in the case of patients with asthma or immune disorders, as examples. It may also be fruitful to use this pre-made diagram for clarity or ease of use. We hope it quickly recapitulates the clearest points from the literature review and incorporates other ways in which—especially habitual—marijuana use may impact functioning.

Summary and Conclusions

For quick reference, outcomes are graded on strength of data below (++++ = strongest data, + = weakest data).

Disease/outcome	Risk of onset	Worsening of course
Psychotic disorders	++++	++
Bipolar and related disorders	++	++++
Depressive disorders	+++	+
Anxiety disorders	++	+
Trauma- and stressor-related disorders	+	++

As has been demonstrated, the intersection of cannabis use and psychiatric outcomes is an area with many opportunities for further exploration. The extant data show clear correlations in the course of some disorders, but not in others. In disorders such as schizophrenia and depression, it appears quite clear that use is tied to earlier onset of symptoms, but other areas require further investigation, such as determining the impact of cannabis use on the development of PTSD. The course and severity of symptoms has also been a frequent target of study. Our literature review shows that mania, depression of both unipolar and bipolar etiologies, and psychoses in general tend to worsen with THC consumption. There is insufficient data to draw strong conclusions about worsening of symptoms in PTSD or anxiety disorders as of this writing.

In addition to exploring the current research, we have also importantly discussed the clinical application of these findings. Translating this information into patient-digestible terms and ideas can mean the difference between a positive clinical outcome or "more of the same."

As will be explored in the next chapter, new data and approaches are being considered and studied for cannabis use disorders when comorbid with other psychiatric pathology—the evaluation and treatment of such patients is discussed in more depth therein. It can be hoped that the data we present, combined with informed evaluation and cutting-edge treatment, may yield better outcomes for all patients for whom we care.

Highlights Box 8.1 Key Points for Patient Psychoeducation

- Cannabis use is strongly associated with earlier onset of schizophrenia and other psychotic-spectrum illnesses.
- The data are less clear for risk of onset of bipolar disorder with cannabis use, although risk for mania is suggested. The course of bipolar disorder symptoms does seem worsened with cannabis use.
- Both risk of onset and earlier age of onset in depressive disorders are increased with cannabis use, but based on limited studies, the course of depression does not seem changed by cannabis use.
- There is a clear association between cannabis use and risk of onset of social anxiety disorder, but the risk for worsened disease course in anxiety disorders or trauma-mediated conditions remains under-studied.
- ADHD and attentional disorders appear to be strongly concurrent with cannabis use, with a prevalence many times that of the general population. The presence of either diagnosis complicates the treatment of both issues.

Highlights Box 8.2 Key Points in Treatment and Management

- Discussing the impacts of cannabis use can be difficult! Patients may have many reasons for use; understanding these reasons is important.
- Focusing on stronger data or known outcomes may help, as can exploring personal impacts specific to the patient.
- Alternatively, reducing harm or use amount/potency may still be admirable treatment targets with some patients.
- Understanding the patient as a person, his or her working relationship with the provider, and the treatment setting are all likely to yield better outcomes.

References

1. National Academies of Sciences Engineering and Medicine, Health and Medicine Division, Board on Population Health and Public Health Practice, Committee on the Health Effects of Marijuana: an Evidence Review and Research Agenda. The health effects of cannabis and cannabinoids: the current state of evidence and recommendations for research. Washington, DC: National Academies Press; 2017. https://doi.org/10.17226/24625.
2. Di Forti M, Marconi A, Carra E, Fraietta S, Trotta A, Bonomo M, et al. Proportion of patients in South London with first-episode psychosis attributable to use of high potency cannabis: a case-control study. Lancet Psychiatry. 2015;2(3):233–8. https://doi.org/10.1016/S2215-0366(14)00117-5.
3. Di Forti M, Quattrone D, Freeman TP, Tripoli G, Gayer-Anderson C, Quigley H, et al. The contribution of cannabis use to variation in the incidence of psychotic disorder across Europe (EU-GEI): a multicentre case-control study. Lancet Psychiatry. 2019;6(5):427–36. https://doi.org/10.1016/S2215-0366(19)30048-3.

4. Starzer MSK, Nordentoft M, Hjorthøj C. Rates and predictors of conversion to schizophrenia or bipolar disorder following substance-induced psychosis. Am J Psychiatry. 2018;175(4):343–50. https://doi.org/10.1176/appi.ajp.2017.17020223.
5. Donoghue K, Doody GA. Effect of illegal substance use on cognitive function in individuals with a psychotic disorder: a review and meta-analysis. Neuropsychology. 2012;26(6):785–801. https://doi.org/10.1037/a0029685.
6. Gibbs M, Winsper C, Marwaha S, Gilbert E, Broome M, Singh SP. Cannabis use and mania symptoms: a systematic review and meta-analysis. J Affect Disord. 2015;171:39–47. https://doi.org/10.1016/j.jad.2014.09.016.
7. Feingold D, Weiser M, Rehm J, Lev-Ran S. The association between cannabis use and mood disorders: a longitudinal study. J Affect Disord. 2015;172:211–8. https://doi.org/10.1016/j.jad.2014.10.006.
8. Pinto JV, Medeiros LS, Santana da Rosa G, Santana de Oliveira CE, de Souza Crippa JA, Passos IC, et al. The prevalence and clinical correlates of cannabis use and cannabis use disorder among patients with bipolar disorder: a systematic review with meta-analysis and meta-regression. Neurosci Biobehav Rev. 2019;101:78–84. https://doi.org/10.1016/j.neubiorev.2019.04.004.
9. Zorrilla I, Aguado J, Haro JM, Barbeito S, López Zurbano S, Ortiz A, et al. Cannabis and bipolar disorder: does quitting cannabis use during manic/mixed episode improve clinical/functional outcomes? Acta Psychiatr Scand. 2015;131(2):100–10. https://doi.org/10.1111/acps.12366.
10. Lev-Ran S, Le Foll B, McKenzie K, George TP, Rehm J. Bipolar disorder and co-occurring cannabis use disorders: characteristics, co-morbidities and clinical correlates. Psychiatry Res. 2013;209(3):459–65. https://doi.org/10.1016/j.psychres.2012.12.014.
11. Hasin DS, Sarvet AL, Meyers JL, Saha TD, Ruan WJ, Stohl M, et al. Epidemiology of adult DSM-5 major depressive disorder and its specifiers in the United States. JAMA Psychiat. 2018;75(4):336–46. https://doi.org/10.1001/jamapsychiatry.2017.4602.
12. Lev-Ran S, Roerecke M, Le Foll B, George TP, McKenzie K, Rehm J. The association between cannabis use and depression: a systematic review and meta-analysis of longitudinal studies. Psychol Med. 2014;44(4):797–810. https://doi.org/10.1017/S0033291713001438.
13. Feingold D, Rehm J, Lev-Ran S. Cannabis use and the course and outcome of major depressive disorder: a population based longitudinal study. Psychiatry Res. 2017;251:225–34. https://doi.org/10.1016/j.psychres.2017.02.027.
14. Kessler RC, Petukhova M, Sampson NA, Zaslavsky AM, Wittchen H-U. Twelve-month and lifetime prevalence and lifetime morbid risk of anxiety and mood disorders in the United States: anxiety and mood disorders in the United States. Int J Methods Psychiatr Res. 2012;21(3):169–84. https://doi.org/10.1002/mpr.1359.
15. Hser Y-I, Mooney LJ, Huang D, Zhu Y, Tomko RL, McClure E, et al. Reductions in cannabis use are associated with improvements in anxiety, depression, and sleep quality, but not quality of life. J Subst Abus Treat. 2017;81:53–8. https://doi.org/10.1016/j.jsat.2017.07.012.
16. Kedzior KK, Laeber LT. A positive association between anxiety disorders and cannabis use or cannabis use disorders in the general population--a meta-analysis of 31 studies. BMC Psychiatry. 2014;14:136. https://doi.org/10.1186/1471-244X-14-136.
17. Botsford SL, Yang S, George TP. Cannabis and cannabinoids in mood and anxiety disorders: impact on illness onset and course, and assessment of therapeutic potential. Am J Addict. 2020;29(1):9–26. https://doi.org/10.1111/ajad.12963.
18. Wilkinson ST, Stefanovics E, Rosenheck RA. Marijuana use is associated with worse outcomes in symptom severity and violent behavior in patients with posttraumatic stress disorder. J Clin Psychiatry. 2015;76(09):1174–80. https://doi.org/10.4088/JCP.14m09475.
19. Carpentier PJ, Levin FR. Pharmacological treatment of ADHD in addicted patients: what does the literature tell us? Harv Rev Psychiatry. 2017;25(2):50–64. https://doi.org/10.1097/HRP.0000000000000122.

20. Notzon DP, Pavlicova M, Glass A, Mariani JJ, Mahony AL, Brooks DJ, Levin FR. ADHD is highly prevalent in patients seeking treatment for cannabis use disorders. J Atten Disord. 2020;24(11):1487–92. https://doi.org/10.1177/1087054716640109.
21. Whiting PF, Wolff RF, Deshpande S, Di Nisio M, Duffy S, Hernandez AV, et al. Cannabinoids for medical use: a systematic review and meta-analysis: a systematic review and meta-analysis. JAMA. 2015;313(24):2456–73. https://doi.org/10.1001/jama.2015.6358.

Evaluation of Co-occurring Psychiatric Disorders and Cannabis Use in the Outpatient Setting

9

Sirish Veligati and Alexis Ritvo

Clinical Case

James is a 53-year-old male veteran with a history of chronic bronchitis who presents to an outpatient psychiatric clinic due to progressively worsening irritability that has led to conflict at work. He reports symptoms including depressed mood, anhedonia, hopelessness, irritability, chronic anxiety, sleep onset disturbance due to racing anxious thoughts, and always feeling "on edge." He works as a car salesman, but is now at risk of losing his job because he has on several occasions unexpectedly lashed out verbally at his customers. He attributes the onset of his symptoms to his divorce 6 years ago, though he is guarded about details of his marital discord. Since then, he has undergone two separate trials of SSRIs, prescribed by his primary care provider, with minimal improvement. On the other hand, he reports that "smoking weed is the only thing that helps" with his anxiety. He had heard that cannabis was a natural, nonaddictive, alternative medicine for depression and anxiety, and he has been smoking daily for a few years now.

Introduction

Patients like James frequently present to the outpatient psychiatric clinic, complaining of unremitting psychological distress in the setting of escalating cannabis use. While some patients explicitly use cannabis to seek relief from their symptoms, many only intermittently use cannabis on a recreational basis. Between these two ends of the spectrum, however, lie many patients who engage in varying degrees of problematic cannabis use without consideration that cannabis may be driving their psychopathology. As such, it falls to the psychiatrist to not only screen their patients

S. Veligati (✉) · A. Ritvo
Department of Psychiatry, University of Colorado School of Medicine, Denver, CO, USA
e-mail: sirish.veligati@cuanschutz.edu; alexis.ritvo@cuanschutz.edu

P. Riggs, T. Thant (eds.), *Cannabis in Psychiatric Practice*, Psychiatry Update 3,
https://doi.org/10.1007/978-3-031-04874-6_9

for substance use, but to gather more detailed information about the history of their symptoms and their cannabis use, discerning how cannabis may be impacting the trajectory of mental health. Translating this information into clinical practice can be challenging, as increasing public acceptance of cannabis as "medicine" can lead to conflicts in shared decision-making. Clinician attitudes themselves can further complicate matters, as they often vary greatly based on state cannabis legalization status and the practitioner's cultural background. Given this broad diversity of attitudes, it is not only critical to ascertain a comprehensive assessment of the patient's cannabis use, but to do so in a nonjudgmental fashion that maintains the therapeutic alliance. This chapter will review best practices for assessing a patient's cannabis use pattern, detecting underlying use disorders, correlating it with lifelong psychiatric history, and setting the stage for treatment of problematic cannabis use while simultaneously enhancing therapeutic rapport.

Review of Literature

Opening the Conversation: Broaching the Topic of Cannabis While Building Rapport

Given increasing prevalence of use particularly among young adults [1], combined with a trend of decreasing perceived harm [2], it is recommended to query history of recent cannabis use among all patients in the outpatient psychiatric setting. This often involves administering a general substance use screening tool such as the ASSIST (see Table 9.1) to patients prior to their intake appointment. However, some clinicians feel that this is unnecessarily in-depth for all comers and subjects patients to evaluation fatigue. As such, cannabis use is often revealed during the first interview with a new provider. This initial discussion of cannabis can set the stage for the patient–physician relationship; thus it is critical to minimize the patient's experience of judgment while establishing credibility as a well-versed authority on cannabis. A few brief and tactful questions can detect red flags for problematic use patterns, prompting a more extensive evaluation later on in the interview.

A simple but powerful means of transitioning from the history of present illness to substance use may sound like the following: "Many patients struggling with your symptoms use substances to help themselves feel better. Do you use cannabis? And if so, how often?" This efficient transition from psychiatric symptoms to substance use both normalizes the patient's experience and demonstrates the provider's experience with patients using cannabis. When working with self-conscious patients that may respond poorly to such direct questioning, it can be helpful to introduce the topic by querying how their support network uses or relates to cannabis. One such example is in the 5P's approach to substance use screening for pregnant women, a very vulnerable population, which involves a progressive discussion of their peers', partner's, parents', past, and finally present substance use behavior [3].

After briefly screening for regular cannabis use, it is recommended to transition into their positive motivations for use, phrasing questions nonjudgmentally to

Table 9.1 Cannabis use screening and assessment tools

Instrument	Description	Items
Cannabis Use Disorder Identification Test (CUDIT) [9]	– 10 items – Past 6 months	• Frequency of use • Typical duration "stoned" • Failed attempts to stop • Failing to meet expectations • Concentration impairments • Frequency of extended intoxication • Withdrawal-related use • Guilt or remorse • Cannabis-related injuries • Peers expressing concern
CUDIT-Revised [10]	– 8 items – Past 6 months – Shorter that CUDIT – More closely resembles DSM-5 cannabis use disorder criteria	• Frequency of use • Typical duration "stoned" • Failed attempts to reduce or stop • Failing to meet expectations • Concentration impairments • Time spent acquiring, using, or recovering • Physically hazardous use • Personal consideration to reduce or stop
Cannabis Abuse Screening Test (CAST) [11]	– 6 items – Lifetime history – Better suited for social consequences in adolescence – Does not gauge amount or frequency	• Using cannabis before midday • Using cannabis alone • Social problems • Memory problems • Peers expressing concern • Failed attempts to reduce or stop
Alcohol, Smoking, and Substance Involvement Screening Test (ASSIST) [12]	– 71 items total – Queries 11 drug categories (including IV drug use) – Comprehensive but efficient and easy to interpret – NIDA developed a free online modified version: https://archives.drugabuse.gov/nmassist	• Lifetime use history • Past 3 month use frequency • Urges to use • Health/social/legal/financial consequences • Failing to meet expectations • Peers expressing concern • Unsuccessful attempts to reduce

strengthen rapport early in the interview. For example, asking "why do you use cannabis?" can place patients in a defensive stance, whereas "what does smoking marijuana help you with?" can be remarkably disarming for patients. This approach reassures patients that the clinician is openly curious rather than dismissive, and it validates patients' behaviors without necessarily condoning them. Common motivations for use include "it's the only thing that lets me feel happy" or "it's how I shut off my brain after work," and they usually reveal other underlying psychiatric symptoms. Maintain an attentive ear for symptoms like sleep disturbance, pain, anxiety, depression, and auditory hallucinations. Orienting treatment plans toward these symptoms usually helps address both the presenting complaint and problematic cannabis use.

This nonjudgmental approach to cannabis use serves many functions simultaneously. Clinicians can efficiently gauge the extent of the patient's cannabis use, establish credibility as a provider familiar with cannabis, expand upon the patient's psychiatric complaints, and validate the patient's experience of suffering. Adopting this patient-centered clinical attitude not only prepares the patient for more detailed evaluation as needed, it also fosters a positive and trusting patient–clinician relationship.

Gathering Details: Diagnosing Underlying Substance Use Disorder

While the information gathered thus far can influence treatment plans and build rapport, it is insufficient for detecting the presence of an underlying cannabis use disorder. Note that a history of recent or current cannabis use does not automatically indicate a use disorder, even in regions where cannabis remains legally prohibited. Similarly as with alcohol, some patients may partake in consumption well within social (if not legal) norms and without experiencing harmful consequences of addiction. However, if the patient's briefly-described use does raise concern for a use disorder, the clinician must further explore the contextual picture of their consumption. This typically involves a significant amount of information gathering and may require frequent redirection to stay on track. Listen for signs that the patient has failed to meet social obligations, experienced consequences from use, developed physiological tolerance, and/or struggled to reduce their use. These features broadly define DSM-5 criteria for cannabis use disorder [4], and thoroughly eliciting this information during initial evaluations can critically inform the patient's treatment course.

The first step in evaluating for cannabis use disorder involves characterizing the amount of cannabis being consumed. Unfortunately, there is no standardized dose of cannabis in the way that there exists a standardized "drink" of alcoholic beverages. However, it remains useful to gauge a general idea of how much cannabis patients are consuming. Start by reviewing a list of common routes—bowls, bongs, joints, blunts, dabs, vapes, or edibles—to elicit the patient's typical pattern. Naming these routes of consumption explicitly indicates credibility by demonstrating an understanding of common terminology. For patients consuming commercially produced edibles, THC content is typically advertised in milligrams per dose. For those smoking cannabis flower, however, it is helpful to understand the quantity consumed in terms of the number of bowls, joints, or blunts smoked per day. Alternatively, clinicians can ask how frequently the patient purchases cannabis, and how much they typically purchase in ounces or grams. Note that cannabinoid concentration in cannabis products today is substantially higher than cannabis grown during the past several decades [5]. Measuring amounts consumed is significantly more difficult when patients consume high-potency THC concentrates like waxes and dabs [6]. Nonetheless, given that these products are associated with higher risk of psychosis [7], it is important to identify the extent of their use. Helpful questions may include the type of concentrate they are using, its potency (i.e., percent THC), how they use it (e.g., torch or vape pen), and how many "hits" they will take during a typical period of use. Once the amount and frequency of cannabis use is established, further questions should explore whether the patient has experienced symptoms of tolerance, withdrawal, and loss of control of their use. For instance, have they ever tried to reduce or stop their use in the past? If yes, how did they feel and how long were they able to reduce or stop for?

Many of the criteria for cannabis use disorder involve the patient's social context when they consume cannabis. Do they typically smoke alone or with other people? What activities does the patient prefer while using cannabis? How might their peers describe their behavior change while intoxicated? How would they describe their relationship with cannabis? These questions ease patients into discussing social consequences of cannabis use. Have their friends or family members expressed concern about the extent of their substance use? Is the patient concerned about living up to their responsibilities? Along these lines, it is important to explicitly ask about occupational consequences. Has the patient presented to work while intoxicated, or received reprimands from supervisors lately? While the presence of legal consequences is no longer an explicit criteria for substance use disorders in the DSM-5, repeated legal consequences are considered a social consequence. These commonly include DUIs, issues with distributing or growing cannabis, or other related encounters with law enforcement.

Diving into the details of the patient's current use pattern can clarify the presence of an underlying cannabis use disorder, but the work does not end there. Regular cannabis use interacts with psychiatric symptoms in complex ways, and the clinician must deepen their inquiry to apprehend the root cause of the patient's distress. Capturing a lifelong history of both the patient's mental health and substance use is often necessary to discern accurate diagnoses and create a strong foundation for treatment planning.

Chicken or Egg: Correlating Psychiatric History and Cannabis Use History

Pushing beyond the presence of a current use disorder, exploring the patient's lifetime history of cannabis use, psychiatric symptoms, and physiologic symptoms can reveal important diagnostic information. Gathering longitudinal history can clarify which of the patient's complaints should be attributed to underlying psychopathology as opposed to substance-related distress. Frequently, these features strongly correspond with one another in ways that patients do not initially recognize, and this process can help patients gain new perspective into how cannabis is affecting their life.

To gather a lifetime history, clinicians can begin by asking open-ended questions about the patient's first use of cannabis, periods they used regularly, and periods of highest frequency use. Historically, cannabis use throughout the lifetime has been limited by access, with higher periods of use during college or military service.

However, this is dramatically changing as recreational cannabis legalization spreads in popularity. It is important to inquire about any extended periods of significant reduction or abstinence, and how social and psychological aspects of the patient's life might have changed during that period. Exploring the patient's past psychiatric history is quite similar to a typical psychiatric evaluation, but take note of how their psychiatric symptoms relate temporally to their substance use history. For example, many patients will begin to use cannabis after developing intolerable anxiety or insomnia, whereas other patients will describe struggling with worsening depressive symptoms or paranoia after they begin cannabis use. It can be useful to explicitly draw a timeline with the patient that illustrates their pattern of cannabis use as well as periods of persistent psychiatric symptoms.

The impact of cannabis use on the patient's health can be difficult to elicit directly, as patients are commonly under the popular impression that cannabis is entirely safe and nonaddictive. However, cannabis withdrawal syndrome has now been formally identified as a diagnosis in DSM-5, including psychiatric symptoms like irritability, restlessness, sleep disturbance, and physical symptoms like headache, abdominal discomfort, and sweating [4]. Providing psychoeducation about cannabis withdrawal syndrome sometimes provides validation and relief for patients that have failed attempts to reduce their consumption. Other physical symptoms of chronic cannabis use include respiratory symptoms, risk of injury, and possible cardiometabolic effects [8]. Drawing complaints from earlier portions of the evaluation can help prompt a discussion of side effects, tolerance, and withdrawal symptoms. Such an example with James may proceed, "I hear that you're struggling with high anxiety and irritability throughout the workday, only finding relief from cannabis when you return home. These symptoms sound similar to cannabis withdrawal. How do you think these might be related?" Not only does this present an opportunity to educate patients, but orienting the discussion in this fashion also plants seeds of ambivalence to be elicited later on during treatment with motivational interviewing strategies.

Highlights Box 9.1 Evaluating Cannabis Use During the Interview

- *Initial Screening*
  - Screen all patients for cannabis use.
    - See Table 9.1 for selected screening instruments.
  - Adopt a nonjudgmental approach that emphasizes rapport-building.
    - University of Missouri-Kansas City School of Nursing and Health Studies has a useful Screening, Brief Intervention, and Referral to Treatment (SBIRT) program with many resources including a free 3.5-hour SBIRT training.
    - https://www.sbirt.care/training.aspx
  - Explore the patient's motivations for use, setting the stage for behavioral interventions discussed in Chap. 10.

- *Assessing for Cannabis Use Disorder*
  - Become familiar with typical names, routes (flower, edibles, etc.), amounts, and costs of cannabis.
    - A helpful open-source resource that includes social, scientific, and anecdotal articles about cannabis https://www.erowid.org/plants/cannabis/cannabis.shtml
    - A substantial review of current literature on cannabis, geared toward the public https://streetdrugs.org/marijuana/
  - Occasional cannabis use, even if illicit, does not automatically meet criteria for cannabis use disorder.
  - Among higher-risk patients, ensure a complete evaluation of all 12 use disorder criteria. These features will likely not arise during the interview unless the clinician explicitly queries them.
- *Correlating Psychiatric History with Cannabis Use History*
  - Complete a thorough psychiatric review of systems with every patient.
  - Capture the patient's lifetime history of both psychiatric symptoms and cannabis use before anchoring to a diagnosis.
  - Expand the assessment beyond psychiatric illness by also querying common physical symptoms associated with cannabis use and withdrawal.

Formal Screening Instruments

Performing an in-person, comprehensive evaluation is necessary to fully understand how cannabis may be affecting the patient. However, this process can be augmented by implementing formal screening tools in the clinical workflow. These validated screening instruments can be provided to patients prior to an intake evaluation, or following subsequent encounters. They illustrate a rough picture of a patient's use pattern, and they allow for rapid, quantifiable interpretation. Many of the questions directly query criteria for cannabis use disorder by asking about physical dependence (tolerance and withdrawal), loss of control of use, cravings, and consequences (social, physical, and psychological). However, no single assessment queries all 12 criteria of cannabis use disorder, and no tool can gather critical information about the context of the patient's use and symptoms.

Given the direct nature of the questions and lack of a therapeutic environment during completion, some patients may feel threatened or assume a defensive stance as they proceed through the screener. Not only may this lead to minimization and response bias, it may affect the patient's attitude toward treatment before they even first meet with their provider. Between this concern and the fact that these screening tools are specific to cannabis, it may be beneficial to ask patients to complete these assessments after an initial encounter, rather than before. Most importantly, these screening tools provide little information about the patient's lifetime history of cannabis use, as most questions only date back to a maximum of 6 months ago. This aspect of evaluation is especially important, as there is often a complex relationship between patients' psychiatric symptoms, their substance use, and their developmental history. Screening tools can be very helpful for gathering more quantifiable information about patients' cannabis use, but they are no replacement for further exploration during clinical interviews.

Summary and Next Steps

Despite cannabis growing increasingly popular, patients rarely present to their psychiatrist complaining about their cannabis use. It is the duty of the clinician to intentionally screen each patient for cannabis use, detect underlying use disorders, and clarify how cannabis may be impacting their psychiatric complaints. Validated screening instruments can facilitate the evaluation process, but open and in-depth conversation is needed to complete a comprehensive assessment. The presence of cannabis use alone does not meet criteria for cannabis use disorder, but often interacts with the patient's mental health nonetheless. The next chapter examines strategies for managing co-occurring cannabis use and psychopathology, work that often hinges on a well-founded therapeutic alliance. This chapter has delineated recommendations to gather needed information while simultaneously strengthening rapport with the patient, a foundation that will be critical for patients to tolerate the difficult work of managing substance use. Furthermore, the assessment process itself sets the stage for treatment by providing opportunities for psychoeducation and drawing connections that promote the patient's insight into how cannabis use has been affecting their life.

Highlights Box 9.2 Key Points for Patient Psychoeducation

- In addition to widespread legalization, there is a decreasing perception of harm associated with cannabis use, and many patients are not aware that it can be addictive.
- Cannabis use alone does not qualify for cannabis use disorder, even in regions where it is legally prohibited.
- True amounts of cannabis are difficult to quantify given both high variation in routes of consumption and increasing cannabinoid concentrations.
- Cannabis use is associated with many physical consequences of use, including formal recognition of Cannabis Withdrawal Syndrome in the DSM-5.
- Formal screening tools can be effective for collecting quantifiable supplementary data about patient's pattern of cannabis use, but do not replace in-person evaluation.

Highlights Box 9.3 Key Points in Treatment and Management

- Adopt a nonjudgmental approach to evaluating patient's cannabis use, fostering rapport early on by exploring their own motivations for use.
- Become familiar with common terminology, amounts, and routes of administration for cannabis, as this helps to establish credibility.
- Take advantage of opportunities to provide brief psychoeducation during the evaluation of patient's cannabis use and psychiatric history.
- Work with patients while drawing connections between their cannabis use patterns and mental health history, setting the stage for eliciting ambivalence.

References

1. Burns RM, Caulkins JP, Everingham SS, Kilmer B. Statistics on cannabis users skew perceptions of cannabis use. Front Psych. 2013;6(4):138.
2. Carliner H, Brown QL, Sarvet AL, Hasin DS. Cannabis use, attitudes, and legal status in the US: a review. Prev Med. 2017;1(104):13–23.
3. Center for Substance Abuse Treatment. Chapter 4: Screening and assessment. In: Substance abuse treatment: addressing the specific needs of women. Rockville (MD): Substance Abuse and Mental Health Services Administration (US); 2009. Treatment Improvement Protocol (TIP) Series, No. 51. Available from: https://www.ncbi.nlm.nih.gov/books/NBK83253/. Accessed: 29 June 21.
4. American Psychiatric Association. Diagnostic and statistical manual of mental disorders. 4th ed. American Psychiatric Association: Arlington, VA; 2013.
5. Cascini F, Aiello C, Di Tanna G. Increasing delta-9-tetrahydrocannabinol (Δ-9-THC) content in herbal cannabis over time: systematic review and meta-analysis. Curr Drug Abuse Rev. 2012;5(1):32–40.
6. Mariani JJ, Brooks D, Haney M, Levin FR. Quantification and comparison of marijuana smoking practices: blunts, joints, and pipes. Drug Alcohol Depend. 2011;113(2–3):249–51.
7. Murray RM, Englund A, Abi-Dargham A, Lewis DA, Di Forti M, Davies C, Sherif M, McGuire P, D'Souza DC. Cannabis-associated psychosis: neural substrate and clinical impact. Neuropharmacology. 2017;15(124):89–104.
8. National Academies of Sciences, Engineering, and Medicine. The health effects of cannabis and cannabinoids: the current state of evidence and recommendations for research. Washington, DC: The National Academies Press; 2017. https://doi.org/10.17226/24625.
9. Adamson SJ, Sellman JD. A prototype screening instrument for cannabis use disorder: the Cannabis Use Disorders Identification Test (CUDIT) in an alcohol-dependent clinical sample. Drug Alcohol Rev. 2003;22(3):309–15.
10. Adamson SJ, Kay-Lambkin FJ, Baker AL, Lewin TJ, Thornton L, Kelly BJ, Sellman JD. An improved brief measure of cannabis misuse: the Cannabis Use Disorders Identification Test-Revised (CUDIT-R). Drug Alcohol Depend. 2010;110(1–2):137–43.
11. Legleye S, Karila L, Beck F, Reynaud M. Validation of the CAST, a general population Cannabis Abuse Screening Test. J Subst Abus. 2007;12(4):233–42.
12. Humeniuk RE, Henry-Edwards S, Ali RL, Poznyak V, Monteiro M. The Alcohol, Smoking and Substance Involvement Screening Test (ASSIST): manual for use in primary care. Geneva: World Health Organization; 2010.

Treatment of Co-occurring Psychiatric Disorders and Cannabis Use in the Outpatient Setting

10

Sirish Veligati and Alexis Ritvo

Introduction

The previous chapter reviewed the approach to clinical evaluation of cannabis use in patients presenting to outpatient psychiatric clinics. Once the clinician has completed the information-gathering phase of the interview, the focus of the visit transitions to the management of the patient's cannabis use in the setting of their other mental health problems. By now, the clinician has determined whether or not the patient's cannabis use currently meets criteria for a use disorder (see DSM-5 criteria for cannabis use disorder presented in Chap. 5). Regardless, the clinician must consider the risks and benefits of the patient's cannabis use in the context of their other psychiatric symptoms and medications, applying their knowledge of how cannabis use affects illness prognosis and outcome. This chapter will review management of comorbid psychiatric conditions, and then explore strategies for reduction of high-risk cannabis use and psychosocial and pharmacological treatments for cannabis use disorder.

Clinical Case

Hannah is a thoughtful 29-year-old, first-generation Asian-American occupational therapist with a history of ADHD who presents to outpatient psychiatry for worsening depression. Hannah began to struggle with inattentive symptoms near the end of elementary school. Suffering grades in middle school

S. Veligati (✉) · A. Ritvo
Department of Psychiatry, University of Colorado School of Medicine, Denver, CO, USA
e-mail: sirish.veligati@cuanschutz.edu; alexis.ritvo@cuanschutz.edu

P. Riggs, T. Thant (eds.), *Cannabis in Psychiatric Practice*, Psychiatry Update 3,
https://doi.org/10.1007/978-3-031-04874-6_10

prompted her parents to have her pediatrician complete a clinical evaluation that confirmed a diagnosis of ADHD and subsequently led to her briefly taking a prescription stimulant with good effect. At 23 years old she presented to her primary care provider for a depressive episode that coincided with extended unemployment after graduating from college, and she was started on an antidepressant. Since then, she reported moderate benefit from the antidepressant, "it allowed me to get out of bed and get through OT school." "It also made me feel numb inside, I couldn't really be happy either," so she self-discontinued her antidepressant after a year.

When asked about her history of substance use, she reported occasional alcohol use during college consisting of one to two beers (standard size can and strength) or a glass of wine 1–2 days per week. She first tried cannabis about 2 years ago at age 27, when she took a few hits from a joint at a party and noticed that it made her feel "happy, relaxed, and bubbly." Approximately 6 months ago, she began regularly buying her own marijuana at a local dispensary, and her consumption escalated to daily use over the course of a few months. Since then, she's noticed decreased motivation to socialize outside work or go to the gym as well as increasing difficulty with sustained attention at work, especially when writing up new patient evaluations. Further evaluation reveals that despite her high frequency of use, Hannah meets criteria for only a mild severity cannabis use disorder.

Review of Literature

Psychoeducation and Harm Reduction

When the clinician begins addressing such a patient's psychiatric complaints, they must first triage management of their cannabis use. This prioritization is based not only on whether the patient meets formal criteria for cannabis use disorder, but also based on the risk of continued cannabis use exacerbating the patient's other psychiatric disorders (as discussed in Chap. 8). Therefore, some cases will warrant a more intensive treatment plan for substance use than others. At minimum, clinicians should seek the patient's permission to provide relevant psychoeducation to all patients using marijuana. This includes general information about independent health effects of both chronic use and withdrawal, in addition to screening and counselling to avoid high-risk physical activities like driving, swimming, bicycling, or skiing/snowboarding while intoxicated [1]. In a more personalized fashion, however, psychoeducation should focus on the risks conferred by continued cannabis use on the patient's comorbid mental illness. Please refer to the highlights box at the end of Chap. 8 for summary of some key points to provide to patients based on their specific comorbid psychopathology.

Highlights Box 10.1 Psychoeducational Resources

- Clinicians working in outpatient mental health settings should provide research-based psychoeducation to patients about the physical and mental health effects associated with cannabis use:
  - CDC provides resources on the health effects of marijuana at www.cdc.gov/marijuana
  - NIDA publishes a Research Report and several DrugFacts on marijuana, including marijuana concentrates and synthetic cannabinoids (K2/spice) at www.drugabuse.gov
  - SAMSHA has developed a helpful resource called "Learn about Marijuana Risks" at www.samhsa.gov/marijuana

After reviewing relevant psychoeducation points, many patients may remain uninterested or feel unable to pursue abstinence. Thus, it is important to develop a collaborative and feasible approach that reduces the risks of continued consumption. This may include monitoring the type, quantity, and frequency of a patient's cannabis use in addition to tracking the corresponding severity of their co-occurring psychiatric symptoms. Another harm reduction approach may include recommendations to avoid high-potency THC products like waxes, dabs, and shatter and—if amenable—trial isolated CBD products rather than THC. For patients suffering from concurrent respiratory symptoms, switching their route of cannabis consumption to edibles and topicals rather than smoking may provide some relief. In each of these situations, the clinician respects the patient's current motivation to change and acknowledges that recommendations toward total abstinence are unlikely to be effective, and may even jeopardize therapeutic alliance. The goal is to minimize the harm associated with ongoing use and optimize the patient's well-being.

Clinical Case

Hannah was struggling with several different psychiatric complaints that modified the prognostic risk associated with her cannabis use. While she endorsed cannabis as "the only thing that lets me feel joy," it is likely that her daily cannabis use contributed to worsening depressive and inattentive symptoms. This information was reviewed with Hannah, who remained skeptical that cannabis could be worsening her depressive symptoms. Nonetheless, she was concerned about its impact on her motivation, inattention, and work performance. Overall, she expressed some worry, but was ambivalent about complete abstinence.

This opened the door for a fuller discussion about how she could reduce the negative impact of her cannabis use on her work. First, Hannah was educated about signs or symptoms of problematic use that she could remain alert for. The cannabis use disorder criteria provided a convenient framework for this topic, with symptoms falling into one of three categories: physical dependence (tolerance or withdrawal), consequences from use (social, occupational, or health-related), and loss of control over use (cravings, urges, unsuccessful efforts to control use, or spending a lot of time obtaining/using/recovering from cannabis). Beyond these criteria, the conversation included recommendations that Hannah track her psychiatric symptoms as well, noting how her mood and attention were affected by changes in her use pattern. Finally, a simple and cursory review of harm reduction strategies left Hannah convinced to "steer clear of waxes and dabs" and curious about isolated CBD products.

Psychosocial Interventions

After having triaged the prognostic risk of the patient's cannabis use, briefly gauged the patient's attitude toward the substance, and appropriately addressed comorbid psychiatric symptoms, the focus of session moves toward fostering behavioral change. The psychosocial interventions with good evidence for helping adults decrease or abstain from cannabis are Motivational Interviewing (MI), Motivational Enhancement Therapy (MET), and combination Cognitive Behavioral Therapy (CBT) with Contingency Management (CM) [1].

Motivational Interviewing (MI) and its operationalized counterpart Motivational Enhancement Therapy (MET) are both highly non-directive strategies that focus on eliciting and then resolving the patient's ambivalence toward their substance use in order to foster behavioral change. Ambivalence refers to the patient's own simultaneous yet conflicting desires to maintain and change their behavior. The role of the physician here is to actively support the patient's self-efficacy by highlighting and exploring their own desire for change. As such, it is critical to adopt a balanced and non-stigmatized attitude toward the patient's cannabis use, as this will foster more accurate information, patient–clinician trust, and decrease defensiveness during later work [2]. Patients can initially present anywhere along a broad range of interest in reducing their consumption. As such, the first step in MI involves identifying where the patient fits along the stages of change, a spectrum derived from the Transtheoretical Model [3] that includes precontemplation, contemplation, preparation, action, maintenance, and relapse.

MET serves as a brief, protocolized MI intervention lasting 1–4 sessions that has demonstrated clinical efficacy comparable to 12-session substance abuse treatment programs [4]. Given the high prognostic risk of cannabis use among patients suffering from psychosis, MI strategies have even been adapted into MET protocols specific for psychotic patients [5]. While these techniques can be helpful for many patients at different stages of change, it is particularly adept for mobilizing patients in precontemplation, contemplation, and planning. During these stages, resolving the patient's ambivalence serves the important function for supporting them into the next stage. MI alone has also shown efficacy in decreasing frequency and quantity of cannabis use in adults [6]. As the patient transitions into the planning, action, and maintenance stages of change, techniques from CBT become increasingly useful.

Clinical Case

Given Hannah's—albeit skeptical—concern about how cannabis use impacted her work life, she fell into the contemplation stage of change. On the one hand, she endorses an acute improvement in her mood symptoms when she smokes marijuana, giving her a brighter, and more hopeful outlook. On the other hand, she worries about how quickly her use frequency escalated to daily, having to hide her substance use from her family, and her worsening work performance. Throughout the interview, explicitly eliciting Hannah's motivations and worries revealed that she felt risks of ongoing use outweighed the benefits she endorsed. She was hopeful that starting a new antidepressant medication, bupropion, would provide her with the energy and motivation to partake in work without leading to feelings of "numbness" that she previously experienced with SSRIs. Near the end of this encounter, she declared openly that she was planning to dedicate conscious effort to maintaining abstinence, thus demonstrating a transition from contemplation into the planning stage of change.

CBT is an evidence-based, time-limited treatment modality that has proven efficacy for a broad range of psychiatric complaints. While the formal therapy protocol usually involves regular meetings over a 12-week course, utilizing the tenets and approach of CBT more flexibly can provide benefit in the outpatient psychiatric setting as well. When applied to substance use in particular, the clinician and patient work together to examine the thoughts, feelings, and behaviors that surround the patient's cannabis use. In this way, it is particularly helpful for patients that have transitioned past contemplation stage, into the planning, action, maintenance, and relapse stages of change. This exploration calls for a very detailed appraisal of the motivations, triggers, cravings, and internal stimuli that precede use. See Highlights Box 10.2 for recommended training resources for the above psychosocial treatments.

As discussed in Chap. 5, contingency management is another evidence-based treatment effective for substance use disorders. As a reminder, contingency management is a behavioral therapy in which individuals receive rewards to provide immediate positive reinforcement for evidence of positive behavioral change [7]. While there is strong evidence for its use in adolescents with cannabis use disorder, the evidence has not been as well replicated for adults [8]. A clinical environment that specializes in treating substance use disorders and other co-occurring psychiatric disorders may be better equipped to develop a robust contingency management protocol. However, utilizing strategies related to contingency management can be useful in the office setting, particularly when working with patients who would benefit from treatment with controlled substances, and also partake in heavy marijuana use.

With the increased risk of misuse, dependence and diversion of controlled prescription medications such as stimulants, benzodiazepines, and Z-drugs, clinicians may prescribe these controlled substances on the condition that a patient demonstrates ability to significantly cut back or abstain from high-risk use of substances, including cannabis. As discussed in Chap. 8, untreated ADHD is often associated with high levels of impulsivity and comorbid substance use. As such, if a patient has ADHD, it is critical to address these underlying symptoms with an appropriate regimen, which—in the case of moderate to severe symptoms—often includes prescription stimulants. Adequately treating underlying ADHD may increase the likelihood that a patient will be able to reduce or abstain from substances including cannabis. While a history of prescription medication misuse or substance use disorder warrants discretion when considering stimulant medications, occasional cannabis use alone is not a contraindication to prescribing a stimulant. Particularly given dramatically increasing social acceptance of cannabis, this may be compared to the notion of refraining to provide a stimulant medication based on a history of occasional alcohol use. Nonetheless, safer alternatives to stimulants, like bupropion and atomoxetine, may be good first-line treatment options for patients that exhibit a concerning pattern of cannabis use and remain in the precontemplation stage of change.

Many patients struggling with anxiety endorse using cannabis to manage their anxiety, and some present to psychiatric clinics seeking benzodiazepines. Unlike the case with prescription stimulants for ADHD, benzodiazepines are not the standard of care for long-term treatment of anxiety disorders. Comorbid regular cannabis use, particularly when motivated by anxiety complaints, is a concerning feature that demands caution when considering initiation of a benzodiazepine. Independent of the physiological hazards of these medications, they often foster an externalized locus of control that worsens prognosis. On the other hand, if a patient is requesting a small supply of benzodiazepines to be used for very specific circumstances, such as fear of flying, and endorses only occasional social use of cannabis, then prescribing a benzodiazepine may be reasonable. In all cases however, close monitoring of the patient's underlying complaints, cannabis use, and medication filling patterns should be employed to ensure appropriate utilization of the medicine.

In treating patients who exhibit a markedly concerning pattern of cannabis use that contraindicates treatment with a controlled substance, clinicians may offer the prescription on the condition that the patient can demonstrate a substantial reduction in marijuana use. Urine samples can be collected periodically to track creatinine-adjusted THC metabolite levels, which can reveal trends in cannabis use patterns while accounting for the patient's level of hydration [9, 10]. Ongoing provision of controlled medications can be made contingent upon the patient demonstrating longitudinally that they can quit or significantly cut back to occasional use (less than daily use or no more than three times per week) of lower potency cannabis. Patients should be advised to abstain for at least 24 h prior to providing a sample as recent use will cause an acute elevation of the THC metabolite level. If the patient is unable to demonstrate a downtrend in their creatinine-adjusted THC metabolite level, then it may be reasonable to establish participation in a higher level of substance use treatment as the condition for continued prescription. Keep in mind that while conditional prescribing may be appropriate in some circumstances, general psychiatric treatment itself should be offered to all patients, regardless of their motivation for change.

Clinical Case

Hannah had previously reported a diagnosis of ADHD in middle school with a good response to a prescription stimulant. She denies any history of prescription medication abuse, diversion, or selling illicit drugs, and her regular cannabis use onset fairly recently. Inadequately treated ADHD symptoms are likely to increase her risk of problematic substance use and impede her ability to significantly cut back or abstain from marijuana. It would be reasonable to discuss with her a conditional trial of a prescription stimulant if bupropion proves insufficient.

Highlights Box 10.2 Psychosocial Treatment Resources

Clinicians working in outpatient mental health settings should access evidence-based psychosocial treatments

- MI and MET
  - SAMSHA Treatment Improvement Protocol (TIP) Series No. 35 on Enhancing Motivation for Change in Substance Use Disorder Treatment https://store.samhsa.gov/product/TIP-35-Enhancing-Motivation-for-Change-in-Substance-Use-Disorder-Treatment/PEP19-02-01-003 PCSS SUD 101 Curriculum. Module 9: Principles of Motivational Interviewing: Useful for Primary Care Physicians. https://pcssnow.org/education-training/sud-core-curriculum/
  - PCSS Motivational Enhancement Techniques: Working with Patients with Substance Disorders or High Risk Using (1 hr., free, registration required) https://pcssnow.org/event/motivational-enhancement-techniques-working-with-patients-with-substance-disorders-or-high-risk-using/
- CBT-SUD
  - VA CBT-SUD manual [11] https://www.treatmentworksforvets.org/wp-content/uploads/2018/04/CBT-SUD-Therapist-Manual.pdf
  - VHA TRAIN CBT-SUD Online Training (1 h, free, registration required) https://www.va.gov/COMMUNITYCARE/docs/providers/VHA_TRAIN.pdf
  - CBT4CBT is a self-guided web-based program that teaches CBT skills for substance use disorders that has been well studied and can be used to supplement a clinician's treatment https://cbt4cbt.com/

Pharmacologic Options

While the above behavioral strategies represent the mainstay of treating comorbid cannabis use, medications can play an adjunctive role for those struggling with behavioral strategies alone. As of this writing, there are no FDA-approved pharmacologic treatments for cannabis use disorder. However, a fair amount of research has explored potentially promising options.

Many of these medications help decrease risk of relapse via one of two mechanisms. Some medications address the patient's underlying psychiatric symptoms—such as anxiety or insomnia—that perpetuates their cannabis use, while other medications mitigate the negative effects of cannabis withdrawal [12]. Cannabis withdrawal is poorly recognized in the public sphere, and it was not recognized as a syndrome until DSM5. Brief psychoeducation about the symptoms associated with this syndrome—irritability, aggression, anxiety, depressed mood, restlessness, sleep difficulty, and decreased appetite or weight loss—can help many patients characterize why they struggle with craving or relapse.

Gabapentin demonstrated promising preliminary evidence of efficacy in treatment of cannabis use disorder and withdrawal. During a 12-week randomized placebo-control trial of adults with cannabis use disorder, treatment with gabapentin 1200 mg was associated with significant reductions in cannabis use (both frequency and amount), withdrawal symptoms, cravings, sleep disturbance, and depression scores, in addition to improved measures of executive functioning [13]. Since then, however, preliminary results from a larger and more fully powered controlled trial have revealed contradicting evidence that suggest gabapentin is not effective for decreasing use [14].

In small trials, naltrexone, an opioid receptor antagonist, has shown evidence for decreasing the reinforcing effect of cannabis [15], and the extended-release injectable naltrexone helped individuals significantly decrease their cannabis use days-per-week [16]. However, larger controlled clinical trials of naltrexone for cannabis use disorder are needed. Nonetheless, for patients exhibiting high-risk alcohol use or alcohol use disorder, naltrexone may also help them significantly decrease or abstain from alcohol use.

In addition to those mentioned above, there are several other medications that have been investigated for their efficacy in reducing cannabis use or withdrawal symptoms. Of note, a trial of N-acetylcysteine in adults did not show decreased cannabis use [17] like it had in a previous study with adolescents [18]. Some of these have included several SSRIs, atypical antidepressants (e.g., mirtazapine, nefazodone, bupropion), atomoxetine (specifically among adults with comorbid ADHD), buspirone, lithium, and valproic acid; however, these trials are far from definitive. While some evidence reveals a reduction in withdrawal symptoms with cannabinoid agonists, like nabilone, dronabinol, nabiximols, and epidiolex, these drugs have not demonstrated efficacy for reducing cannabis use [19–22]. Unfortunately, the limited evidence for these medications suggests that they are largely ineffective for this indication [23]. That being said, it is important to keep in mind that treatment of the patient's underlying psychiatric comorbidity remains a key aspect of their care. Frequently, underlying mood, anxiety, attentional, and even psychotic disorders lead to symptoms that drive patients' cannabis use, and these medications can be highly effective in the appropriate context. A parallel effort toward managing the patient's underlying psychopathology, while also providing behavioral and pharmacologic interventions to support their reduction in cannabis use, is vital to pave the way for a hopeful prognosis.

Clinical Case

When Hannah followed up a few weeks after initiating bupropion, she felt more energized, less depressed, and more durably focused throughout her workday. She had reduced her cannabis use substantially, but still found herself smoking a few times a week after struggling with cravings following a stressful workday. She especially noted difficulty sleeping on nights she did not smoke. To decrease Hannah's risk of returning to heavy, daily marijuana use, next steps in treatment targeted her poor sleep and cravings.

Some simple options to improve her sleep included low dose trazodone or mirtazapine. Regarding her cravings, Hannah was informed about a program offering CBT-SUD sessions to specifically target her cannabis use. Adjunctively, she was offered a trial of naltrexone to see if it helped with cravings. She was educated about the medication's effect on opioid agonists, particularly relevant for acute injuries. She expressed interest in giving naltrexone a try, and was instructed to start with 25 mg at bedtime with a snack and—if tolerating—increase to 50 mg after 6 days. Hannah was very receptive to this explanation, and left our office hopeful about this new medication.

Finally, if she is unable to control her use or quit cannabis, despite optimum management of her co-occurring psychiatric symptoms, Hannah warrants referral to specialty addiction treatment. This can include an addiction-trained therapist or even intensive outpatient treatment options. In the case that this higher level of treatment is needed, it remains critical that her outpatient psychiatrist coordinate with the addiction specialist(s) and continue to manage her psychiatric medications.

Summary and Next Steps

This chapter has delineated an approach to managing patients' cannabis use in the outpatient psychiatric setting. The foundation of this management relies on the adoption of a MI-informed, non-confrontational, and non-stigmatized attitude while evaluating the patient's cannabis use history. Building on an established therapeutic rapport, the clinician must then triage their efforts based on both the patient's use pattern and the prognostic risk conferred by cannabis use on the patient's comorbid psychiatric illness. All patients should be provided with individualized psychoeducation. For patients with limited interest in changing their behaviors, clinicians may review harm reduction strategies and implement conditional prescribing practices with controlled substances. Regarding the latter strategy, keep in mind that a patient's insistence to use cannabis is not sufficient justification to refrain from providing psychiatric care, but does call for caution when prescribing medications with risk for physical dependence, misuse and/or addiction. On the other hand, patients expressing interest in behavioral change are likely to benefit from practices derived from MI, to explore and resolve their ambivalence toward cannabis use. Others that find themselves struggling with the threat of relapse may benefit from CBT to engage in a rigorous examination of the thoughts, feelings, and behaviors surrounding their cannabis use, Finally, there are several promising—albeit preliminary—pharmacologic options to support patients' pursuit of abstinence, such as gabapentin and naltrexone. With relatively small adjustments to clinical practice, starting with evaluation and persisting in treatment, clinicians have the ability to dramatically decrease the negative impact of cannabis use on their patients' lives.

Highlights Box 10.3 Key Points for Patient Psychoeducation

- MI has shown efficacy in decreasing frequency and quantity of cannabis use in adults.
- The psychosocial treatments with the most evidence for treating cannabis use disorder in adults are CBT, MI, and MET.
- Cannabis use alone is not a contraindication to treatment of ADHD with a stimulant and may warrant conditional prescribing practices. Untreated ADHD is a strong risk factor for substance use disorders.
- There are no FDA-approved medications for the treatment of cannabis use disorder.

Highlights Box 10.4 Key Points in Treatment and Management

- Develop a targeted approach to managing patients' cannabis use that incorporates prognostic risk, severity of use, and readiness for change.
- Regardless of the patient's readiness to change their cannabis use, offer to provide every patient individualized psychoeducation about the impacts of cannabis use.
- Utilize strategies from MI as the mainstay treatment approach to promote the patient's own desire and self-efficacy for behavior change.
- Collaborate with patients to develop feasible goals along a spectrum from harm reduction to complete abstinence.
- Pharmacologic interventions should target the underlying psychiatric symptoms and cannabis withdrawal symptoms that motivate the patient's cannabis use.

References

1. Hartman RL, Huestis MA. Cannabis effects on driving skills. Clin Chem. 2013;59(3): 478–92.
2. Latchford G, Duff A. A brief guide to motivational interviewing. Clinical Psychology Training Programme, Leeds Institute of Health Sciences, University of Leeds. 2010.
3. DiClemente CC, Schlundt D, Gemmell L. Readiness and stages of change in addiction treatment. Am J Addict. 2004;13(2):103–19.
4. Project MATCH Research Group. Matching alcoholism treatments to client heterogeneity: project MATCH three-year drinking outcomes. Alcohol Clin Exp Res. 1998;22(6):1300–11.
5. Bonsack C, Montagrin Y, Favrod J, Gibellini S, Conus P. Motivational interviewing for cannabis users with psychotic disorders. L'encephale. 2007;33(5):819–26.
6. Calomarde-Gómez C, Jiménez-Fernández B, Balcells-Oliveró M, Gual A, López-Pelayo H. Motivational interviewing for cannabis use disorders: a systematic review and meta-analysis. Eur Addict Res. 2021;7:1–5.
7. Petry NM, Alessi SM, Olmstead TA, Rash CJ, Zajac K. Contingency management treatment for substance use disorders: how far has it come, and where does it need to go? Psychol Addict Behav. 2017;31(8):897.
8. Gates PJ, Sabioni P, Copeland J, Le Foll B, Gowing L. Psychosocial interventions for cannabis use disorder. Cochrane Database Syst Rev. 2016;(5):CD005336.
9. Huestis MA, Blount BC, Milan DF, Newmeyer MN, Schroeder J, Smith ML. Correlation of creatinine-and specific gravity-normalized free and glucuronidated urine cannabinoid concentrations following smoked, vaporized, and oral cannabis in frequent and occasional cannabis users. Drug Test Anal. 2019;11(7):968–75.
10. Dominion Diagnostics [Internet]. Understanding elimination patterns with creatinine adjusted drug values. Dominion Diagnostics. [Cited 2021 June 30]. Available from: https://www.dominiondiagnostics.com/education/understanding-elimination-patterns-creatinine-adjusted-drug-values
11. DeMarce JM, Gnys M, Raffa SD, Karlin BE. Cognitive behavioral therapy for substance use disorders among veterans: therapist manual. Washington, DC: U.S. Department of Veterans Affairs; 2014.
12. Budney AJ, Vandrey RG, Hughes JR, Thostenson JD, Bursac Z. Comparison of cannabis and tobacco withdrawal: severity and contribution to relapse. J Subst Abus Treat. 2008;35(4):362–8.
13. Mason BJ, Crean R, Goodell V, Light JM, Quello S, Shadan F, Buffkins K, Kyle M, Adusumalli M, Begovic A, Rao S. A proof-of-concept randomized controlled study of gabapentin: effects on cannabis use, withdrawal and executive function deficits in cannabis-dependent adults. Neuropsychopharmacology. 2012;37(7):1689–98.
14. Mason BJ, The Scripps Research Institute. Gabapentin treatment of cannabis dependence. In: ClinicalTrials.gov [Internet]. Bethesda, MD: U.S. National Library of Medicine; 2009 Sept 10 [last updated 2010 Jun 6; results first received 2010 Jun 6; cited 2021 Jun 30]. Available from: http://clinicaltrials.gov/show/NCT00974376 ClinicalTrials.gov Identifier: NCT00974376.
15. Haney M, Ramesh D, Glass A, Pavlicova M, Bedi G, Cooper ZD. Naltrexone maintenance decreases cannabis self-administration and subjective effects in daily cannabis smokers. Neuropsychopharmacology. 2015;40(11):2489–98.
16. Notzon DP, Kelly MA, Choi CJ, Pavlicova M, Mahony AL, Brooks DJ, Mariani JJ, Levin FR. Open-label pilot study of injectable naltrexone for cannabis dependence. Am J Drug Alcohol Abuse. 2018;44(6):619–27.
17. Gray KM, Sonne SC, McClure EA, Ghitza UE, Matthews AG, McRae-Clark AL, Carroll KM, Potter JS, Wiest K, Mooney LJ, Hasson A. A randomized placebo-controlled trial of N-acetylcysteine for cannabis use disorder in adults. Drug Alcohol Depend. 2017 Aug;1(177):249–57.
18. Gray KM, Carpenter MJ, Baker NL, DeSantis SM, Kryway E, Hartwell KJ, McRae-Clark AL, Brady KT. A double-blind randomized controlled trial of N-acetylcysteine in cannabis-dependent adolescents. Am J Psychiatr. 2012;169(8):805–12.

19. Levin FR, Mariani JJ, Pavlicova M, Brooks D, Glass A, Mahony A, Nunes EV, Bisaga A, Dakwar E, Carpenter KM, Sullivan MA. Dronabinol and lofexidine for cannabis use disorder: a randomized, double-blind, placebo-controlled trial. Drug Alcohol Depend. 2016;1(159):53–60.
20. Levin FR, Mariani JJ, Brooks DJ, Pavlicova M, Cheng W, Nunes EV. Dronabinol for the treatment of cannabis dependence: a randomized, double-blind, placebo-controlled trial. Drug Alcohol Depend. 2011;116(1–3):142–50.
21. Allsop DJ, Copeland J, Lintzeris N, Dunlop AJ, Montebello M, Sadler C, Rivas GR, Holland RM, Muhleisen P, Norberg MM, Booth J. Nabiximols as an agonist replacement therapy during cannabis withdrawal: a randomized clinical trial. JAMA Psychiat. 2014;71(3):281–91.
22. Trigo JM, Soliman A, Quilty LC, Fischer B, Rehm J, Selby P, Barnes AJ, Huestis MA, George TP, Streiner DL, Staios G. Nabiximols combined with motivational enhancement/cognitive behavioral therapy for the treatment of cannabis dependence: a pilot randomized clinical trial. PLoS One. 2018;13(1):e0190768.
23. Nielsen S, Gowing L, Sabioni P, Le Foll B. Pharmacotherapies for cannabis dependence. Cochrane Database Syst Rev. 2019;(1):CD008940.

Acute Intoxication and Agitation/Violence

11

Scott A. Simpson and Peter Gooch

Clinical Case

A 25-year-old male is brought to the emergency department (ED) by police and ambulance for agitation and violence. He destroyed a television set and punched a hole in the wall during an argument with his parents, with whom he lives. When you see him, the patient is anxious about being seen in the ED and incurring a bill, stating "I don't have insurance." He is a combat veteran, has never had mental health treatment, and smokes cannabis daily to manage anxiety and insomnia. "It's the only thing that keeps me level." He denies other substance use, psychosis, or mood symptoms. The psychiatry team calls the patient's parents, who report that since the patient was dishonorably discharged 3 years ago, he has not had regular employment or a romantic relationship. "All he does is play video games in our basement and smoke pot." They say he is highly irritable, stays up all night and sleeps during the day, and occasionally demonstrates strange behaviors that make no sense, like repeatedly re-arranging objects. "Today I told him he needs to get a job, and he blew up. He is always unpredictable and angry," his mother explains, "and I want to help, but I don't feel safe with him at home." His mother further shares that sometimes she hears the patient talking to himself. The patient dismisses his parents' concerns, saying "I'm 25, of course I get upset when they tell me what to do. They don't understand what it's like to have this anxiety. I tried working, but it was too much." There is no clear temporal correlation between cannabis use and violence from either the patient or his mother. The patient had a citation for driving while intoxicated on alcohol last year. The court suggested he pursue mental health treatment, although the patient declined the need for services at that time.

S. A. Simpson (✉)
Behavioral Health Services, Denver Health and Hospital Authority, Denver, CO, USA
e-mail: scott.simpson@dhha.org

P. Gooch
Goucher College, Baltimore, MD, USA

P. Riggs, T. Thant (eds.), *Cannabis in Psychiatric Practice*, Psychiatry Update 3,
https://doi.org/10.1007/978-3-031-04874-6_11

Introduction and Literature Review

Cannabis use is common among patients presenting in the ED and is involved in more than 2.7 million ED visits each year [1]. ED patients with complications of cannabis use are disproportionately young, male, non-Hispanic Black or Hispanic, uninsured, and economically marginalized [2]. This population is at high risk for using other substances of abuse and having a co-occurring mental health diagnosis [3]. In fact, up to half of cannabis-associated ED presentations are related to mental health effects of acute use—these effects include anxiety, mood symptoms, psychosis, aggression, and violent behavior [2].

The clear association between tetrahydrocannabinol (THC) and violence risk has long been observed in laboratory and clinical studies. This relationship is mediated through multiple neurotransmitters, including endocannabinoids, and THC's adverse impacts on psychosis, mood, impulsivity, and cognition [4]. THC's association with violence risk is apparent among myriad clinical populations. For example, patients' use of cannabis is a stronger predictor of violence after discharge from psychiatric hospitalization than the use of either alcohol or cocaine [5], and cannabis use is associated with worse symptom control and more frequent violent behavior among veterans with posttraumatic stress disorder (PTSD), as could be suspected in this clinical case [6]. There may be a dose–response relationship between more frequent cannabis consumption and the likelihood of perpetrating violence [7]. Studies have repeatedly demonstrated that cannabis use predicts violent behavior among youth, intimate partners, and patients with serious mental illness, independent of other psychiatric and substance use disorders [4, 8–10]. Aggressive behavior may be particularly common during either active use or withdrawal, when cognitive and emotional impairments related to THC are particularly pronounced [11].

The clinical case described at the start of this chapter is thus typical in terms of patient characteristic and circumstance. ED visits for violence during cannabis intoxication occur but are relatively rare [2]. More common are presentations like this case in which, while the patient has a cannabis use disorder, acute intoxication is unclearly timed with the event precipitating the ED visit. This young male patient has multiple potential comorbidities including PTSD, alcohol use disorder, and gaming addiction. These other conditions impact the patient's violence risk, too. An approach to acute management, disposition planning, and risk assessment must weigh all these co-occurring symptoms and morbidities.

Limitations persist in our understanding of the relationship between cannabis use and violence. The use of large diagnosis-based datasets probably understates the prevalence of cannabis-related ED visits, although bias towards diagnosing cannabis use disorder in the context of its complications could overstate the frequency of cannabis use's most severe manifestations. It is difficult to estimate the dose–response relationship between cannabis use and risk, particularly as new THC products (e.g., shatter, resin) have become available since legalization. The frequent presence of comorbid disorders and demographic factors make confounding a frequent challenge in interpreting data.

Medical and Psychiatric Symptoms of Intoxication

Initial treatment in the emergency setting must include ensuring patient and staff safety and identification of the patient's intoxication as the cause of agitation when applicable. Cannabis is a highly lipophilic drug with a rapid onset of action and slow hepatic metabolism. Cannabis intoxication occurs within 2 h of cannabis use and is characterized by tachycardia, dry mouth, conjunctival injection, and increased appetite. Perceptual disturbances and psychosis may occur; some intoxicated patients are highly anxious or paranoid. The drug's pharmacokinetics and toxidrome vary substantially based on route of cannabis administration, co-occurring substance use and medical conditions, and individual variations in metabolism. Because THC remains present in the body for weeks after administration during chronic use, urine toxicology screening has little role in determining the timing of cannabis use and presence of intoxication; serum blood levels are rarely available in clinical settings.

Cannabis intoxication may also result in agitation, a syndrome of motoric hyperactivity and restlessness. Agitation is an emergent condition for which quick diagnosis and management is crucial for averting dangerous outcomes. Agitation has many possible causes: metabolic disturbances (e.g., hypoglycemia, hyponatremia), hypoxia, traumatic brain injury, peri-ictal phenomena, infectious delirium, or intoxication and withdrawal syndromes related to other substances. No trials describe specific treatments for acute cannabis-induced agitation. As with treatment for all agitation, patients should first be offered trauma-informed verbal de-escalation. Oral benzodiazepines are considered first-line treatment, and oral second-generation antipsychotics may be considered for patients with accompanying psychosis [12]. Patients unable to remain safe may require constant observation and/or a low stimulation environment in order to reduce the risk of restraint, seclusion, or involuntary medication administration.

Medical risks of acute intoxication are primarily cardiovascular [13]. Increased sympathomimetic tone may cause hypertension and cardiac complications. Because cannabis users are prone to hypokalemia, there is an increased risk of arrhythmias. An electrocardiogram should be obtained, and telemetry should be considered for patients with a known cardiac history. Patients with a history of pulmonary conditions may be at risk for bronchospasms and hypoxia. Other medical sequelae may result from concurrent ingestions. Table 11.1 summarizes the symptoms of cannabis intoxication.

Managing Ongoing Violence Risk

In the clinical case example, having ensured the patient's and staff's acute safety, the clinician may evaluate the patient's ongoing risk for violence in the presence of multiple concerning symptoms. Given the prominence of cannabis use in this presentation, a closer interview may well reveal the characteristic clinical syndrome of

Table 11.1 Signs, symptoms, and complications of cannabis intoxication

Psychiatric	Agitation Anxiety Cognitive impairment Delusions Hallucinations Sleep disturbances
Somatic	Arrhythmias Bronchospasm and wheezing Conjunctival injection Dry mouth Myocardial infarction Tachycardia

cannabis use disorder, in which the patient experiences a range of impairments related to uncontrolled cannabis use [14].

The patient's mental status exam and history suggest the presence of psychosis: disorganized behavior, hallucinations, and perhaps negative symptoms of avolition and alogia. Cannabis use may induce these symptoms or exacerbate pre-existing psychotic illness such as schizophrenia or bipolar disorder [15]. The patient's high premorbid functioning at this age as an active duty combatant suggests against primary psychosis. On the other hand, his dishonorable discharge could reflect historical complications related to the onset of psychosis, problematic substance use, or complex PTSD. Definitive diagnostic determinations are likely impossible within the timeframe of an emergency visit; serial assessments on an outpatient basis will be necessary.

The possible presence of comorbid PTSD and/or alcohol use disorder all inform the clinicians' violence risk assessment in this case and may inform potential treatment recommendations [16]. Other considered diagnoses include concurrent depression, personality pathology, or developmental crisis evidenced by the patient's inability to sustain employment and meaningful relationships during this life stage. In this acute presentation where multiple overlapping diagnoses are possible, the clinician should keep in mind two tenets: (1) Definitive diagnoses may not be possible or necessary in this emergent setting, and (2) Substance treatment will be a necessary component of any reasonable treatment plan regardless of the ultimate formulation. Table 11.2 summarizes modifiable and unmodifiable risk factors related to violence risk in patients with cannabis use disorder.

The confluence of law enforcement and cannabis-related behavioral emergencies is also notable. A review in Washington state found that while legalization decreased the number of marijuana-related arrests, marijuana was still involved in over 40% of police-involved traffic incidents [17]. Police are also likely to be involved in incidents related to violent behavioral emergencies. These encounters pose a risk of fatal outcomes [18]. Mitigating the risk of such community-based violence is an important goal of clinical treatment planning.

Table 11.2 Selected risk factors for violence in patients with cannabis use disorder

Unmodifiable risk factors	Comorbid illness History of self-harm History of perpetrating violence Male sex Younger age
Dynamic/modifiable risk factors	Access to weapons Comorbid substance use Decompensated symptom burden of comorbid illness Frequency and quantity of substance use Intoxication/withdrawal Irritability Psychosis Threatening statements

Treatment Approach

Engaging this patient in substance treatment is likely the single most important intervention for reducing his risk of ongoing violence, and a multimodal behavioral health intervention can prepare this patient for discharge [19]. Specific interventions in this case should include lethal means counseling to secure firearms and medications in the home. Family and friends should be involved in mitigating these risks whenever possible. Clinicians should help the patient develop a behavioral crisis plan that identifies precipitants for the day's events and identifies alternative coping skills such as the use of mindfulness or distraction techniques.

Follow-up care should include one of several evidence-based strategies for treating problematic cannabis use (refer to Chap. 7 for more in-depth review of these strategies). Cognitive-behavioral therapy, contingency management, or motivational enhancement therapy reduce the quantity and frequency of cannabis use behaviors as well as reduce the severity of cannabis dependence symptoms. These approaches are more effective when used in combination [20, 21]. Psychotherapy referrals and/or treatment with medication for any comorbid mental disorders may also be appropriate. Follow-up instructions should be as specific as possible and include an appointment time and hand-off whenever possible [22]. In cases where the patient continues to make threats towards others, the clinician may have a legal duty to warn identified targets or police depending on jurisdiction.

For a variety of reasons, including the natural course of addiction and cultural acceptance of cannabis use, many patients have difficulty accepting that cannabis use may drive problematic psychiatric or medical symptoms. Emergency settings are a unique venue in which the opportunity arises to provide frank psychoeducation to patients, given the often dramatic and dangerous circumstances that bring patients to care. Adverse impacts of cannabis should be contextualized within the patient's own self-reported goals. For instance, does this patient want a job and money? To avoid jail time for violence? If so, how is cannabis impacting those goals? A motivational interviewing approach may be helpful, although limited evidence supports this modality's use for reducing cannabis use. Family may also welcome education on the course of cannabis use disorder, should be validated if necessary in setting healthy boundaries related to their involvement in the care plan, and invited to partner in the care plan. For example, families might attend an outpatient appointment or go to a recovery support group meeting with the patient. Psychotherapeutic interventions may be more effective for younger adults and those without serious mental illness [23]. It is unknown whether a reduction in overall cannabis use or harm reduction would be as effective as abstinence for reducing this patient's violence risk.

Clinicians should always consider the role of higher levels of residential and inpatient care as part of a substance treatment plan. Substance treatment is often guided by the American Society of Addiction Medicine's placement criteria [24]. These criteria suggest higher levels of care based on the risks of withdrawal, psychiatric and medical comorbidities, and recovery environments. Cannabis withdrawal is not medically dangerous, but a patient exhibiting recurrent violence due to cannabis use and who is unable to maintain sobriety in an outpatient setting may require treatment in more acute settings.

Finally, any assessment of the risk of violence towards others should include assessment of the risk of violence towards oneself, i.e., the risk of self-harm and suicide. Suicide risk assessment in the context of cannabis use is covered in Chap. 10 Suicide.

Conclusion

Cannabis use is correlated with violence, both during acute intoxication and over the course of chronic use. Management of violence risk should address not only the cannabis use disorder but also any co-occurring disorders and access to lethal means. Brief interventions may reduce the risk of violence and enhance the likelihood of recovery.

Highlights Box 11.1 Key Points for Patient Psychoeducation

- Cannabis is associated with increased violence risk. This risk is often understated by persons with cannabis use disorder.
- Presentations for cannabis-related complications to ED are common.
- Individuals admitted to the ED with complications of cannabis are more likely than other patients to have another mental health disorder diagnosis.
- No evidence supports specific interventions for reducing the risk of violence among patients with cannabis use disorder.

Highlights Box 11.2 Key Points in Treatment and Management

- Violence risk should be assessed in patients presenting with cannabis-related disorders.
- While violence may occur during cannabis intoxication, many presentations of violence are more nuanced, involving demographic risk factors and comorbid illness amidst chronic cannabis use.
- Cannabis intoxication carries acute medical and psychiatric risks. These risks include cardiovascular complications and agitation.
- No evidence supports specific treatments for cannabis-related agitation. Existing guidelines suggest that oral benzodiazepines are first-line treatments followed by oral antipsychotics.
- Behavioral interventions that reduce access to lethal means and increase the likelihood of ongoing care are beneficial for ameliorating the future risk of violence.

References

1. Zhu H, Wu LT. Trends and correlates of cannabis-involved emergency department visits: 2004 to 2011. J Addict Med. 2016;10(6):429–36.
2. Salas-Wright CP, Carbone JT, Holzer KJ, Vaughn MG. Prevalence and correlates of cannabis poisoning diagnosis in a national emergency department sample. Drug Alcohol Depend. 2019;204:107564.
3. Hall KE, Monte AA, Chang T, Fox J, Brevik C, Vigil DI, et al. Mental health-related emergency department visits associated with cannabis in Colorado. Acad Emerg Med. 2018;25(5):526–37.
4. Dellazizzo L, Potvin S, Athanassiou M, Dumais A. Violence and cannabis use: a focused review of a forgotten aspect in the era of liberalizing cannabis. Front Psych. 2020;11:567887.
5. Dugre JR, Dellazizzo L, Giguere CE, Potvin S, Dumais A. Persistency of cannabis use predicts violence following acute psychiatric discharge. Front Psych. 2017;8:176.
6. Wilkinson ST, Stefanovics E, Rosenheck RA. Marijuana use is associated with worse outcomes in symptom severity and violent behavior in patients with posttraumatic stress disorder. J Clin Psychiatry. 2015;76(9):1174–80.
7. Norstrom T, Rossow I. Cannabis use and violence: is there a link? Scand J Public Health. 2014;42(4):358–63.
8. Dellazizzo L, Potvin S, Dou BY, Beaudoin M, Luigi M, Giguere CE, et al. Association between the use of cannabis and physical violence in youths: a meta-analytical investigation. Am J Psychiatry. 2020;177(7):619–26.
9. Beaudoin M, Potvin S, Giguere CE, Discepola SL, Dumais A. Persistent cannabis use as an independent risk factor for violent behaviors in patients with schizophrenia. NPJ Schizophr. 2020;6(1):14.
10. Johnson RM, LaValley M, Schneider KE, Musci RJ, Pettoruto K, Rothman EF. Marijuana use and physical dating violence among adolescents and emerging adults: a systematic review and meta-analysis. Drug Alcohol Depend. 2017;174:47–57.
11. Guo S, Biegel DE, Johnsen JA, Dyches H. Assessing the impact of community-based mobile crisis services on preventing hospitalization. Psychiatr Serv. 2001;52(2):223–8.
12. Wilson MP, Pepper D, Currier GW, Holloman GH Jr, Feifel D. The psychopharmacology of agitation: consensus statement of the American association for emergency psychiatry project Beta psychopharmacology workgroup. West J Emerg Med. 2012;13(1):26–34.

13. Bui QM, Simpson S, Nordstrom K. Psychiatric and medical management of marijuana intoxication in the emergency department. West J Emerg Med. 2015;16(3):414–7.
14. American Psychiatric Association. Diagnostic and statistical manual of mental disorders: DSM-5. 5th ed. Arlington, VA: American Psychiatric Association; 2013.
15. Marconi A, Di Forti M, Lewis CM, Murray RM, Vassos E. Meta-analysis of the association between the level of cannabis use and risk of psychosis. Schizophr Bull. 2016;42(5):1262–9.
16. Zhai ZW, Hoff RA, Howell JC, Wampler J, Krishnan-Sarin S, Potenza MN. Differences in associations between problematic video-gaming, video-gaming duration, and weapon-related and physically violent behaviors in adolescents. J Psychiatr Res. 2020;121:47–55.
17. Stohr MK, Willits DW, Makin DA, Hemmens C, Lovrich NP, Stanton DL, et al. Effects of marijuana legalization on law enforcement and crime: final report. Washington, DC: National Criminal Justice Reference Services; 2020. Available from: https://www.ojp.gov/pdffiles1/nij/grants/255060.pdf
18. Fuller D, Lamb H, Biasotti M, Snook J. Overlooked in the undercounted: the role of mental illness in fatal law enforcement encounters. 2016.
19. Simpson SA, Monroe C. Implementing and evaluating a standard of care for clinical evaluations in emergency psychiatry. J Emerg Med. 2018;55(4):522–9.e2.
20. Winters KC, Mader J, Budney AJ, Stanger C, Knapp AA, Walker DD. Interventions for cannabis use disorder. Curr Opin Psychol. 2021;38:67–74.
21. National Institute on Drug Abuse. Available treatments for marijuana use disorders. 2020 [cited 2020 July].
22. Smith TE, Haselden M, Corbeil T, Wall MM, Tang F, Essock SM, et al. Effect of scheduling a post-discharge outpatient mental health appointment on the likelihood of successful transition from hospital to community-based care. J Clin Psychiatry. 2020;81(5)
23. Halladay J, Scherer J, MacKillop J, Woock R, Petker T, Linton V, et al. Brief interventions for cannabis use in emerging adults: a systematic review, meta-analysis, and evidence map. Drug Alcohol Depend. 2019;204:107565.
24. Mee-Lee D. American Society of Addiction Medicine. The ASAM criteria: treatment for addictive, substance-related, and co-occurring conditions. 3rd ed. Chevy Chase: American Society of Addiction Medicine; 2013. xv, 460 p

Cannabis and Psychosis

12

Ina Becker and Ryan E. Lawrence

Case

Charles is a 19-year-old college student who is brought to the Emergency Department by his parents after he began acting bizarrely at home. In early life, Charles had an uncomplicated pregnancy followed by normal development. He had no significant medical history aside from mild, exercise induced asthma. He began smoking cannabis intermittently when he was 15 years old. Initially, he smoked at parties with friends. He did not like drinking alcohol and liked the calming effect cannabis had on his social anxiety. Towards the end of high school, he began smoking more regularly "to calm his nerves." He had always been an honor roll student during school and he felt social pressure to get into an elite university. He was accepted to an excellent university, but did not thrive in the competitive environment at the school. He withdrew more into himself, spent more time "studying" alone in his room, and smoked cannabis daily. He bought the cannabis from a peer who praised the cannabis as "some of the strongest stuff available." Halfway through his freshman year he called his parents, asking them to pick him up. He "could not handle being singled out and scrutinized by all the other students." His parents learned that he had been missing classes and not finishing his coursework. Once at home, he continued to spend most of his time alone in his room, and continued to smoke cannabis daily. He taped his windows shut and covered them with towels because, "I don't want the police watching me anymore." At times, he seemed internally preoccupied, talking to himself and

I. Becker · R. E. Lawrence (✉)
Department of Psychiatry, Columbia University Medical Center, New York, NY, USA

Comprehensive Psychiatric Emergency Program, New York-Presbyterian Hospital, New York, NY, USA
e-mail: ib58@cumc.columbia.edu; rel2137@cumc.columbia.edu

P. Riggs, T. Thant (eds.), *Cannabis in Psychiatric Practice*, Psychiatry Update 3,
https://doi.org/10.1007/978-3-031-04874-6_12

gesturing without any apparent context. His self-care began to suffer. He showered once a week and then spent 2 h in the bathroom. His sleep schedule reversed. He went to sleep at 5 am, slept through most of the day, and then stayed up most of the night. He stopped eating regularly. He stopped calling friends. He wrote long multi-page documents of undecipherable text that seemed meaningful to him. When he told his parents that he was afraid someone was trying to kill him, they took him to the Emergency Department for evaluation. During the evaluation, the family reported that Charles has an uncle with schizophrenia.

Introduction

While much public discourse has focused on the purported benefits of cannabis and related products, evidence has been steadily accumulating for an association between cannabis use and the development of schizophrenia and other psychotic disorders. This has been discussed in the medical literature for many years, but it has received limited public attention, causing many individuals and their families to be surprised when it occurs [1].

Table 12.1 Longitudinal cohort studies suggesting an association between cannabis use and psychosis

Swedish Conscript Study	A dose–response relationship was observed between cannabis use by age 18 and schizophrenia by age 45. There was a threefold increase in risk among persons who used cannabis more than 50 times by age 18
Dunedin Birth Cohort Study	Cannabis use by age 15 was associated with an increased risk of schizophreniform disorder at age 26 (odds ratio 11.4)
Dutch Netherlands Mental Health Survey and Incidence Study	Cumulative cannabis use was associated with incident psychotic outcomes measured 3 years later
California Hospital Study	There was an association between hospital admission diagnosis of cannabis use disorder and risk of later hospitalization for schizophrenia (odds ratio 8.16)
Christchurch Health and Development Study	There was an association between cannabis dependence and psychotic experiences
Early Developmental Stages of Psychopathology Study	Any cannabis use at baseline was associated with psychotic symptoms 42 months later
Epidemiological Catchment Area Study	Daily cannabis use was associated with increased risk of psychotic experiences
National Psychiatric Morbidity Survey	An association was found between cannabis dependence and incident psychotic symptoms 18 months later (only in the unadjusted analysis)
Zurich Study	During 30 years of follow-up, cannabis use was associated with schizophrenia symptoms (only in the unadjusted analysis)
Avon Longitudinal Study of Parents and Children	Cumulative cannabis use at age 16 was associated with psychotic experiences at age 18 (result was not significant after adjusting for cigarette use and other illicit drug use)

Source: Gage et al. [2]

Prevalence and Epidemiology

Over the past few decades, studies have consistently found an increased risk of psychosis among heavy cannabis users, daily users, and users with a family history of a psychotic illness in a first degree relative. The risk seems to be dose-related, with more cannabis use leading to a higher risk for psychosis [2, 3].

Large cohort studies have generated much of the evidence for this association (Table 12.1). The first such work was carried out in Sweden in the 1980s, where over 50,000 military recruits were followed longitudinally. Cannabis consumption was identified as a predictor of psychosis, and the amount consumed appeared to be related to the risk of developing schizophrenia. The same cohort was re-analyzed in 2002 and the same dose–response relationship was detected again, with higher amounts of cannabis used and use at a younger age leading to a worsened risk of developing psychosis. The odds ratio for developing schizophrenia was 2.2 among persons who ever used cannabis, and 6.7 for those who had used cannabis more than 50 times [4].

It is not yet clear why some cannabis users develop psychosis and others do not. Individuals with a family history of schizophrenia seem to have an increased risk, as do people who begin cannabis use at a younger age, suggesting that cannabis use acts as an environmental stressor that, combined with other risk factors (e.g., genetic, developmental), promotes the onset of psychosis [5].

Additional evidence for a link between cannabis and psychosis comes from the recent popularity of synthetic cannabinoids, sometimes called "spice" or "K2." While the specific chemical structures of these agents can vary, they function as full agonists of the CB1 cannabinoid receptor. This differs from tetrahydrocannabinol (THC) and endogenous cannabinoids, which are partial agonists. Case reports and case series have reported many instances of persons who use these agents presenting to hospitals with acute florid psychotic symptoms, suggesting a clear link between CB1 receptor activation and psychosis [3, 6].

While providing powerful and compelling evidence for an association between cannabis use and psychosis, these observational studies fall short of proving a causal link [2]. Skeptics note that correlation is not causation. Cannabis could be a marker for unmeasured factors, rather than the cause itself. In multiple studies, adjusting for covariates attenuated and sometimes eliminated the observed association between cannabis and psychosis. Studies relying on self-reports about cannabis use (frequency, quantity, potency) are vulnerable to recall bias and social desirability bias. Longitudinal studies invariably suffer from attrition and sample drift over time. Additionally, there is literature suggesting cannabis use should be viewed as precipitating psychotic symptoms in vulnerable individuals (lowering the age of symptom onset by approximately 5 years), rather than causing the psychotic illness [7].

The association between cannabis use and psychosis has significant implications for public health, given the large numbers of people who use cannabis. In 2013, 9.5% of the population of the USA used cannabis and 2.9% met diagnostic criteria for cannabis use disorder [8].

Importantly, the prevalence of cannabis use in the USA has increased over the last 2 decades, in part because many states have enacted medical marijuana laws, or have legalized recreational use of cannabis and related products. States that have legalized cannabis have found increased use among various age groups beginning with teenagers as young as 13, up through older people. Cannabis use among college students specifically has measurably increased in states that legalized recreational use [8, 9].

Along with the increased prevalence of cannabis use, there has also been—over the last several decades—an increase in the potency of cannabis and related products. The "grass" or "weed" used in the 1960s and 1970s typically contained less than 4% THC and often the same percentage of cannabidiol (CBD). In contrast, many preparations in use today contain upwards of 60% THC, and products containing 90% THC can be purchased legally in some areas. THC is psychotomimetic (capable of inducing psychotic symptoms), while CBD is believed to possess antipsychotic and neuroprotective properties [3]. In lower potency products, such as the plant cannabis of the 1960s and 1970s, THC and CBD content are somewhat balanced. In high potency products, which can be found in newer, laboratory-bred varieties, the THC content is much higher than the CBD content, likely increasing the risk of psychotic symptoms [3].

This combination of more widespread use and more potent product availability is concerning, as each factor could contribute to higher rates of schizophrenia and other psychotic disorders in the community.

While much of the existing literature has focused on cannabis use and psychosis risk among adolescents and young adults (consistent with the usual time course for developing a psychotic illness and theories about neurodevelopment and heightened vulnerability), there is some suggestion of a persistent association between cannabis use and psychosis throughout adulthood, at least until age 65 [10].

Overall, epidemiological and observational data indicate that cannabis use is associated with double the risk of developing psychosis. Among frequent users and persons who use high potency products, the risk of psychosis increases sixfold. It has been estimated that approximately 8–14% of schizophrenia cases could be attributed to cannabis use [5]. The public health implications are significant, especially given the increased prevalence of cannabis use, and the increased potency of those products in recent years.

Neurobiology

A precise understanding of how cannabis and cannabinoids might cause psychosis has not yet been determined. Nevertheless, several research pathways and observations are suggestive (Table 12.2).

The endocannabinoid system in the brain is not itself a primarily dopaminergic system. Rather, the endocannabinoid system modulates dopamine transmission via GABA (gamma-aminobutyric acid) and glutamate at various points of interaction in the brain, including the striatum, the midbrain, and afferent terminal inputs onto

Table 12.2 Neurobiological links between cannabis/cannabinoids and psychotic symptoms

The endocannabinoid system in the brain modulates dopamine transmission via GABA and glutamate (dopamine signaling is likely a key factor in psychosis)
In laboratory studies, cannabis and cannabinoids cause symptoms that resemble schizophrenia
THC causes electroencephalogram changes similar to those seen in schizophrenia
Brain MRI studies of cannabis users show findings also seen among persons with psychotic disorders
Several genes involved with dopamine signaling might be associated with increased risk of psychosis among cannabis users

dopamine axon terminals [11]. Overall, it is believed that the endocannabinoid system acts as a filter of afferent input that shapes how incoming information is conveyed onto dopaminergic neurons and their output targets [11].

Given these interactions with the dopamine system, it is not surprising that cannabis and cannabinoids can cause a variety of symptoms that can resemble schizophrenia, a disorder where disrupted dopamine signaling plays a prominent role.

Human laboratory studies using healthy subjects have consistently shown that cannabis, extracts from cannabis (especially THC), and synthetic cannabinoids can temporarily cause symptoms that resemble the positive, negative, and cognitive symptoms seen in schizophrenia [3]. These symptoms are temporary (duration often depends on route of administration) and dose-dependent (symptoms are more intense and more common at higher doses). Positive symptoms include fragmented thinking, disturbances in space and time perceptions, illusions, hallucinations, paranoia, derealization, and depersonalization. Negative symptoms include blunted affect, reduced spontaneity, internal preoccupation, and amotivation. Cognitive deficits involve working and verbal memory.

Electroencephalogram studies have shown P50 gating deficits among persons with chronic psychotic disorders, among healthy subjects who receive THC, and among chronic cannabis users. P50 gating deficits suggest a disruption of the brain's ability to modulate its sensitivity to incoming sensory information [3]. Other electroencephalogram studies have shown that THC administration disrupts gamma band oscillations, and this correlates with psychotomimetic symptoms (neural oscillations in the gamma band are involved with perception, attention, and working memory). Attenuation of neural oscillations in the gamma band has also been seen in persons with psychotic disorders [3].

Structural brain MRI studies have suggested an association between regular cannabis use and lower gray matter volumes in regions that have been implicated in psychosis (hippocampus, amygdala, putamen, prefrontal cortex) [3]. In diffusion tensor imaging studies, which provide an indication of the integrity of white matter tracts, cannabis users (compared to controls) show reduced fractional anisotropy in the superior longitudinal and uncinate fasciculi, the collosum, the fornix, and the thalamic radiation; tracts that also show reduced fractional anisotropy in psychotic disorders [3].

A variety of PET and SPECT studies have endeavored to clarify the effect of cannabinoids on dopamine, with mixed results [3]. While CB1 activation in rodents stimulates neuronal firing of mesolimbic dopamine neurons and elevates striatal dopamine levels, this has been hard to replicate in human studies. Human studies utilizing THC administration have shown some effects on dopamine release, dopamine reuptake, dopamine synthesis, and dopamine transporter availability, but these effects are not as prominent as those found in studies of other addictive substances (e.g., amphetamines) where major deficits in dopamine release and reuptake are reported. Some evidence suggests that chronic cannabis users show decreased striatal dopamine synthesis, which is contrary to what is usually found in acutely psychotic patients [3]. The only responsible conclusion from these mixed findings is that additional research is needed to elucidate the mechanistic links between cannabis use, dopamine signaling, and increased psychosis risk.

Genetic risk factors likely play an important role in determining which cannabis users go on to develop chronic psychotic symptoms [5]. As mentioned earlier, evidence suggests that cannabis use is more likely to lead to schizophrenia among persons with a family history of schizophrenia versus persons with no family history of schizophrenia. While evidence continues to emerge, and some findings are inconsistent in replication studies, at least three genes have attracted interest. The DRD2 gene (involved with post-synaptic dopamine signaling), especially the rs1076560 T allele, is associated with psychotic disorders among cannabis users. The COMT gene (involved with metabolizing dopamine in the prefrontal cortex), especially the Val-158 polymorphism, is associated with psychosis among cannabis users in some studies. A variant of the AKT1 gene (involved with post-synaptic-dopamine signaling), namely the C/C rs2494732 genotype, also seems to increase the risk of psychosis among cannabis users. These findings are suggestive of a gene–environment interaction contributing to schizophrenia risk, and a rare opportunity to modify a schizophrenia risk factor [5].

A variety of observations suggest the adolescent brain may be especially vulnerable to the psychotogenic effects of cannabis (please see Chap. 2 for more information on the neurodevelopmental impact of cannabis). Multiple studies have pointed to a correlation between starting cannabis use at a younger age (especially heavy use during adolescence) and subsequently developing a psychotic disorder [5]. Studies of brain development have found that CB1 receptor levels in the prefrontal cortex and striatum fluctuate during adolescence [12]. Specifically, the adolescent brain shows a rapid, sustained increase in cannabinoid receptor binding, particularly in the striatum, which is approximately reduced by half in early adulthood. Additionally, expression of the gene that produces CB1 receptors is highest during adolescence and gradually decreases by adulthood. Levels of anandamide (an endogenous cannabinoid naturally found in the brain) and fatty acid amide hydrolase (which degrades endogenous cannabinoids, terminating their signal) fluctuate throughout adolescence [12]. Taken together, these observations suggest periods of heightened sensitivity to cannabinoids during adolescent brain development.

While these multiple lines of investigation do not provide a single or straightforward mechanism by which the use of cannabis and related molecules contributes to the onset of a psychotic illness, they do suggest that mechanistic links are plausible and likely.

Clinical Presentations, Diagnoses, and Treatments

When a patient presents with psychotic symptoms and has been using cannabis or related products, as occurred in the case at the beginning of this chapter, the first challenge is to establish the correct diagnosis. The stakes are high, because incorrect diagnoses could lead to inappropriate treatment plans, needlessly exposing some young adults to long-term antipsychotic medication (risking sedation, weight gain, diabetes, and tardive dyskinesia) or needlessly prolonging the duration of untreated psychosis (risking a worse prognosis). Diagnostic criteria are fairly straightforward in theory; however, clinicians can find it pragmatically challenging to obtain the information necessary to apply the criteria.

Acute Intoxication

As mentioned previously, acute intoxication can imitate many of the symptoms seen in schizophrenia and other psychotic disorders [13], including positive symptoms, negative symptoms, and cognitive symptoms. The hallmark of intoxication is that symptoms are transient and resolve within a few hours of cannabis exposure. A paradigmatic example would be someone who experiences paranoia for a few hours after using cannabis for the first time.

Intoxication can be harder to identify when individuals present with psychotic symptoms and have been using cannabis frequently and/or heavily for weeks, months, or years. A few hours after using cannabis, these individuals will still have significant THC levels in their bodies. Among heavy users, THC remains detectable in the blood for up to a month after the last use [14]. Asking the individual to discontinue the cannabis use and following him or her clinically for several days or weeks would facilitate arriving at a diagnosis, but might not be feasible if the individual is reluctant to disclose psychotic symptoms, has limited insight into how cannabis is contributing to those symptoms, is ambivalent about stopping cannabis use, or does not want to engage in psychiatric follow-up.

For the patient in the opening case, if there are no acute safety concerns, if psychiatric hospitalization is not required, and if intoxication is suspected as the diagnosis, it might be reasonable to build the treatment plan around providing psychoeducation about the association between cannabis use and psychosis (educating both the patient and the family), encouraging cessation of cannabis use, and arranging close outpatient follow-up (within a few days) to assess whether symptoms rapidly improve with cessation of cannabis. The patient and his family should be advised about the possibility of cannabis withdrawal if this plan is implemented.

Substance Induced Psychotic Disorder

No clear line separates intoxication from substance induced psychotic disorder [15] or cannabis induced psychotic disorder [16]. The Diagnostic and Statistical Manual of Mental Disorders (DSM-5) criteria require that hallucinations or delusions predominate in the clinical picture, perhaps implying that intoxication or withdrawal does not predominate. The International Statistical Classification of Diseases and Related Health Problems (ICD-11) better conveys the spirit of the diagnosis by explaining, "the intensity or duration of symptoms is substantially in excess of psychotic-like disturbances of perception, cognition, or behavior that are characteristic of cannabis intoxication or cannabis withdrawal." For patients with this diagnosis, symptoms should resolve within a few days of stopping cannabis use; however, symptoms can persist for weeks and can sometimes require antipsychotic medication.

Making this diagnosis has challenges also. If symptoms resolve rapidly, a diagnosis of intoxication is more likely to be considered. If the symptoms persist for days or weeks, outpatient clinicians may wonder if cannabis use has really ceased (urine toxicology may remain positive for weeks after cessation, limiting its value). Emergency department and inpatient clinicians may experience pressure to start an antipsychotic medication, creating uncertainty about whether subsequent improvements are due to cannabis cessation or to antipsychotic medication.

For the patient in the opening case, if the symptoms are assessed to be more severe or more sustained than would be expected from intoxication, then substance induced psychotic disorder should be considered. It would be reasonable to start an antipsychotic medication for this patient, while also providing the same psychoeducation mentioned above. If the patient prefers not to start a medication and plans to stop using cannabis and follow up closely with an outpatient provider, this could also be a reasonable strategy.

When antipsychotic medication is started, clinicians and patients will face uncertainty regarding how long to continue the medication. If psychotic symptoms really were substance induced, then long-term antipsychotic medication is unnecessary and medications should be tapered off. However, clinicians should also keep in mind that approximately 50% of persons who present with cannabis induced psychotic disorder later go on to develop schizophrenia [17]. For many patients, long-term outpatient follow-up is ideal if it can provide ongoing support for abstaining from cannabis and monitoring for any return of psychotic symptoms.

Schizophrenia or Other Chronic Psychotic Disorder

Some patients who use cannabis develop schizophrenia or another chronic psychotic disorder. These individuals will—especially if untreated—experience chronic positive, negative, or cognitive symptoms even if they stop using cannabis. It can be difficult to know from the outset that a cannabis-using individual has developed schizophrenia (rather than a substance induced psychotic disorder or severe intoxication effects), but over time this diagnosis is likely to become clear. The diagnosis is clear if psychotic symptoms occur in the absence of cannabis use. Treatment should follow established guidelines for treating schizophrenia, including medication management, psychotherapy, and supportive services as needed.

The patient in the opening case has an uncle with schizophrenia, increasing the likelihood of a schizophrenia diagnosis. This information could influence the treatment plan towards starting an antipsychotic sooner and continuing the medication for a longer period of time, both important decisions that would need to be discussed with the patient.

For persons with schizophrenia, stopping cannabis use should be a clinical priority. Cannabis has negative effects on the clinical course of schizophrenia, including: greater declines in social functioning, reduced medication adherence, greater loss of brain volume, more depressive symptoms, and higher rates of relapse and hospitalization [18, 19]. Alternatively, evidence shows that among persons who stop using cannabis after a first episode of psychosis, long-term functional outcomes are better and negative symptoms are less severe [20]. Motivational enhancement therapy and cognitive behavioral therapy are both evidence-based techniques that could help individuals reduce or stop using cannabis.

Synthetic Cannabinoid Intoxication

A special diagnostic consideration when evaluating an individual with new psychotic symptoms is whether the person has been using synthetic cannabinoids. Case reports from the literature indicate that synthetic cannabinoids are capable of causing states of severe agitation and psychosis. Clinical presentations rival the degree of psychosis, agitation, and disorganization seen in methamphetamine intoxication. Clinical presentations commonly include: erratic and bizarre behavior, florid psychosis, paranoia, fragmented thought process, auditory and visual hallucinations, severe mood lability, high levels of agitation, and a high risk of violence. Autonomic instability, with symptoms such as fever, tachycardia, and sweating, are also common [6]. When symptoms do not resolve in a few hours, patients often require psychiatric hospitalization for at least 3–4 days while their mental state returns to baseline and the psychosis resolves.

Over the last 10 years, synthetic cannabinoids (e.g., K2, spice) have been found in many countries [21]. Initially designed in laboratories in an effort to develop novel pain medications, their medical use was quickly abandoned. Subsequently, a street market developed. There are now over 70 different types of synthetic cannabinoids available. Most of them are not listed as Schedule 1 controlled substances, in part because regulators have difficulty keeping up with novel formulations [6].

Synthetic cannabinoids are cheap, readily available in some cities, and are not detected on routine urinary drug tests. These factors make them particularly attractive to homeless persons, incarcerated individuals, and many teenagers. Most users are young males, often between the ages of 13–19. In 2012, 11.4% of twelfth grade high school students reported use of synthetic cannabinoids, making it the second leading drug consumed, after natural cannabis [6].

Treatment of synthetic cannabinoid intoxication or substance induced psychotic disorder primarily involves supportive care. Patients should remain in a safe environment and special attention should be paid to ensuring that they take in adequate fluids and food. Sedation is used as needed. First-line medications are the benzodiazepines, both for their calming effects and for their ability to mitigate seizure risk. Antipsychotics are also frequently utilized, with specific drugs chosen according to their side effect profiles. Data are not currently available regarding how long medications should be continued once the acute symptoms resolve. Outpatient substance abuse treatment is especially important to help the person refrain from further use.

Conclusion

Epidemiological data and cohort studies have long shown an association between cannabis use and the development of schizophrenia and other psychotic disorders. Neurobiological research has suggested a number of pathways by which cannabis and cannabinoids might cause psychotic symptoms. Clinically, the co-occurrence of cannabis use and psychotic symptoms makes it more difficult to establish accurate diagnoses and to formulate appropriate treatment plans, and can make chronic psychotic disorders more difficult to treat.

While it is important to emphasize that most individuals who use cannabis and related products do not develop psychotic symptoms, it is equally important to emphasize that some users are significantly increasing their risk of developing a serious mental illness. Likewise, society is at risk of experiencing increased burden of chronic psychotic disorders. As cannabis use gains wider acceptance, there also needs to be an awareness of the risk of psychosis.

Highlights Box 12.1 Key Points for Patient Psychoeducation

- Cannabis use is associated with an increased risk of developing schizophrenia and other psychotic disorders.
- Cannabis use is one of the few schizophrenia risk factors that is modifiable.
- The mechanism(s) by which cannabis use might cause psychosis are still being researched; multiple possible neurobiological pathways have been identified.

Highlights Box 12.2: Key Points in Treatment and Management

- Distinguishing between cannabis intoxication, substance induced psychotic disorder, and schizophrenia and other psychotic disorders can be challenging. Taking a detailed history and providing close follow-up can be invaluable.
- Making an accurate diagnosis is critically important as the diagnosis will affect treatment planning. The risk of unnecessary exposure to antipsychotic medication must be weighed against the risk of allowing prolonged duration of untreated psychosis.
- Among persons with schizophrenia, cannabis use is associated with a more complicated clinical course.

References

1. O'Donnell J, Hughes T, Innes S. Is marijuana linked to psychosis, schizophrenia? It's contentious, but doctors, feds say yes. USA Today. 2019 Dec 15. 2019.
2. Gage SH, Hickman M, Zammit S. Association between cannabis and psychosis: epidemiologic evidence. Biol Psychiatry. 2016;79(7):549–56.
3. Murray RM, Englund A, Abi-Darham A, Lewis DA, Di Forti M, Davies C, et al. Cannabis-associated psychosis: neural substrate and clinical impact. Neuropharmacology. 2017;124:89–104.
4. Pearson NT, Berry JH. Cannabis and psychosis through the lens of DSM-5. Int J Environ Res Public Health. 2019;16:4149.
5. Volkow ND, Swanson JM, Evins AE, DeLisi LE, Meier MH, Gonzalez R, et al. Effects of cannabis use on human behavior, including cognition, motivation, and psychosis: a review. JAMA Psychiat. 2016;73(3):292–7.
6. Deng H, Verrico CD, Kosten TR, Nielson DA. Psychosis and synthetic cannabinoids. Psychiatry Res. 2018;268:400–12.
7. Barnes TRE, Mutsatsa SH, Hutton SB, Watt HC, Joyce EM. Comorbid substance use and age at onset of schizophrenia. Br J Psychiatry. 2006;188(3):237–42.
8. Hasin DS, Saha TD, Kerridge BT, Goldstein RB, Chou SP, Zhang H, et al. Prevalence of marijuana use disorders in the United States between 2001-2002 and 2012-2013. JAMA Psychiat. 2015;72(12):1235–42.
9. Hasin DS, Sarvet AL, Cerda M, Keyes KM, Stohl M, Galea S, et al. US adult illicit cannabis use, cannabis use disorder, and medical marijuana laws: 1991–1992 to 2012–2013. JAMA Psychiat. 2017;74(6):579–88.
10. Leadbeater BJ, Ames ME, Linden-Carmichael AN. Age-varying effects of cannabis use frequency and disorder on symptoms of psychosis, depression and anxiety in adolescents and adults. Addiction. 2019;114:278–93.
11. Covey DP, Mateo Y, Sulzer D, Cheer JF, Lovinger DM. Endocannabinoid modulation of dopamine neurotransmission. Neuropharmacology. 2017;124:52–61.
12. Chadwick B, Miller MM, Hurd YL. Cannabis use during adolescent development: susceptibility to psychiatric illness. Front Psych. 2013;2013(4):129.
13. D'Souza DC, Perry E, MacDougall L, Ammerman Y, Cooper T, Wu Y-T, et al. The psychotomimetic effects of intravenous delta-9-tetrahydrocannabinol in healthy individuals: implications for psychosis. Neuropsychopharmacology. 2004;29(8):1558–72.
14. Mørland J, Bramness JG. Δ9-tetrahydrocannabinol (THC) is present in the body between smoking sessions in occasional non-daily cannabis users. Forensic Sci Int. 2020;309:110188.
15. American Psychiatric Association. Diagnostic and statistical manual of mental disorders. 5th ed. Arlington, VA: American Psychiatric Association; 2013.
16. International Statistical Classification of Diseases and Related Health Problems, 11th ed [Internet]. 2020. https://icd.who.int/browse11/l-m/en#http://id.who.int/icd/entity/816184127. Accessed 10 Jan 2021.
17. Reid S, Bhattacharyya S. Antipsychotic treatment failure in patients with psychosis and comorbid cannabis use: a systematic review. Psychiatry Res. 2019;280:112523.
18. Hadden KL, LeDrew K, Hogan K, Thomas B. Impact of comorbid cannabis use on outcome in first episode psychosis. Early Interv Psychiatry. 2018;12(5):848–55.
19. Schoeler T, Monk A, Sami MB, Klamerus E, Foglia E, Brown R, et al. Continued versus discontinued cannabis use in patients with psychosis: a systematic review and meta-analysis. Lancet Psychiatry. 2016;3(3):215–25.
20. González-Pinto A, Alberich S, Barbeito S, Gutierrez M, Vega P, Ibáñez B, et al. Cannabis and first-episode psychosis: different long-term outcomes depending on continued or discontinued use. Schizophr Bull. 2011;37(3):631–9.
21. Hobbs M, Kalk NJ, Morrison PD, Stone JM. Spicing it up – synthetic cannabinoid receptor agonists and psychosis - a systematic review. Eur Neuropsychopharmacol. 2018;28(12):1289–304.

Self-Harm and Cannabis Use

13

Thom Dunn

Self-harm and suicide are of considerable concern to psychiatrists and others treating mental illness. In 2019 more than 47,500 Americans died by suicide and a million more were estimated to have attempted [1]. Indeed, suicide rates and prevalence of self-harm are steadily increasing in the United States [2, 3] and are at historic highs. Among the many variables associated with self-harm and suicide is substance misuse [4, 5]. Given the prevalence of cannabis use among many demographic groups, it is useful to understand its relationship, if any, with self-harm. This chapter will review the literature regarding self-harm and suicide and cannabis use and includes a case study of 36-year-old man who stabbed himself in the chest while intoxicated on high-potency cannabis.

Paramedics were called to a man who had stabbed himself. They reported finding the patient "in a supine position with a knife in his chest all the way up to the knife handle." His injuries included a lacerated lung, pericardial trauma, a large diaphragm injury, and a through-and-through stomach injury. Urine drug screen was not initially performed upon admission (16 h later, presence of opioid and benzodiazepines were detected. THC was not part of the panel). Psychiatry was called to assess the patient. Mr. C and his wife reported that he was a 36-year-old man who was with a high-functioning executive with a graduate degree. His psychiatric history was significant only for social anxiety managed by his primary care provider with daily citalopram 20 mg and alprazolam 0.5 mg as needed. Neither the patient nor his wife reported depression nor stressors in the days or weeks preceding this event. That evening he reported feeling upbeat and positive. An intermittent cannabis (flower) user, Mr. C decided to unwind that evening by using a legally acquired, high potency form of the drug. Hours later his wife would be awakened to

T. Dunn (✉)
Behavioral Health Services, Denver Health, Denver, CO, USA

Psychological Sciences, University of Northern Colorado, Greeley, CO, USA
e-mail: thom.dunn@unco.edu

P. Riggs, T. Thant (eds.), *Cannabis in Psychiatric Practice*, Psychiatry Update 3,
https://doi.org/10.1007/978-3-031-04874-6_13

"maniacal laughing" from the TV room. She came down to find Mr. C confused and acting strangely. After she left the house to call 911, he stabbed himself in the chest with a large kitchen knife. He said he had no idea what made him stab himself, that it was impulsive, and that in no way he was trying to kill himself.

A growing number of Americans view cannabis as no more harmful than alcohol and its use (either for purported medicinal uses or recreationally) has been legalized in more than half of US states [6]. Legal cannabis procured from a dispensary in particular is often viewed to be even safer than illicit cannabis [7]. However, there are known deleterious effects associated with cannabis use. As highlighted in Chap. 4, psychiatric sequelae have been associated with its use. For example, a 2014 meta-analysis of 31 studies pooling data of more than 100,000 adults found that after controlling for confounds there is a small magnitude association of cannabis use and anxiety [8]. This is noteworthy when considering the gentleman in this chapter's case study. He reported a history of social anxiety that was sufficiently impairing that he would sometimes pre-medicate with a benzodiazepine during social events. This level of anxiety persisted despite regularly taking citalopram. The literature suggests that cessation of cannabis use may be necessary for Mr. C's anxiety to remit. Certainly his safety evaluation becomes more complicated if he chooses to continue to use cannabis. He may get into a vicious cycle of feeling that he needs cannabis to help curb anxiety, yet will always have anxiety as long as he continues its use.

Association between cannabis use and self-harm (including suicide) must be considered in the context of depression. While there is a literature examining the association between cannabis and depression, there are heterogeneous conclusions. For example, Gobbi and colleagues (2019) performed a meta-analysis of 11 studies with more than 23,000 adolescents making a compelling argument that regular cannabis users have an increased risk of developing major depressive disorder and suicidal ideation [9]. These findings are in contrast, however, to a 2012 study involving Swiss conscripts finding no association between cannabis and depression [10]. Such studies are methodologically complicated and it is not surprising there are conflicting findings in the literature. One interpretation of the heterogeneity is that there is sufficient evidence of an association between cannabis use and depression that, particularly for adolescents, those with risk factors for mood disorders should be cautious about its use. Mr. C had no family history of major depressive disorder, nor did he report previous episodes of a major depressive episode.

When directly examining links between suicide and cannabis use, this literature too has mixed findings. For example, returning to the Swiss conscript dataset, a 2018 analysis found no association with cannabis use and self-harm when confounding variables were controlled for [11]. However, there is other quite compelling evidence to the contrary. A 13-year longitudinal study of more than 2000 Norwegian youths found that individuals in their 20s who had 11+ uses of cannabis in the previous year were at nearly a three times higher risk for death by suicide, even after potential confounds were controlled for [12]. A 2019 meta-analysis found a pooled odds ratio of 3.46 when measuring the association between cannabis use and suicide attempts [13]. This may not be surprising as most studies note that cannabis use itself is associated with well-known risk factors for suicide, including lower socio-economic status, abuse and neglect in childhood, as well as other psychiatric comorbidities [14].

It is reasonable to ask whether cannabis use is merely associated with other factors that drive suicidal behavior. In a rigorous study, however, van Ours and colleagues (2013) examined 30 years of data from more than 1200 individuals in a New Zealand birth cohort study [15]. They used a bivariate mixed proportional hazard model to study cannabis use and suicidal ideation. This framework modeled the transitions into cannabis use and into suicidal ideation to form a fully simultaneous system. Using this model, cannabis use is permitted to impact on the onset of suicidal ideation and suicidal ideation is also permitted to impact on cannabis use. The unobserved heterogeneity terms as they correlate with each transition rate then can be measured. The result is a reliable estimate of the **causal** impact of cannabis use on suicidal behaviors as well as examining causal direction. That is, answering the question whether it is cannabis use that drives suicidal behavior, or do individuals experiencing suicidal ideation seek out the substance [15]? From this remarkable analysis, the authors draw several conclusions interesting to psychiatrists and others who treat mental illness. First, there is a causal effect between using cannabis many times a week and suicidal behavior in susceptible men. Earlier and heavier use predict younger age of first suicidal thoughts. Second, in both men and women, suicidal ideation does not lead to increased cannabis use, presumably as a means to cope [15]. Mr. C, in our case, did endorse using cannabis many times a week, but never endorsed suicidal thinking nor previous suicide attempts.

Mr. C, however, had engaged in serious self-harm while intoxicated on high-potency cannabis. There are other cases reported of similar episodes, albeit typically associated with an onset of psychosis. An Italian group reports a man with "massive" cannabis use that led to a psychotic state while intoxicated on cannabis and self-amputation of his penis and testicles [16]. A gruesome French report describes a gentleman without any psychiatric history actively using high-potency cannabis who then attempted to amputate his arm, self-enucleated both eyes, and then impaled himself on a fence before exsanguinating to death [17]. However, in the case of Mr. C, his self-harm presented as being impulsive while intoxicated on high-potency cannabis. Indeed, Escelsior and colleagues (2021) performed a meta-analysis of cannabis and self-harm involving 16 studies and more than 19,000 individuals, concluding that cannabis use and self-harm are related and theorize that it is increased *impulsivity* during intoxication that can make some users dangerous [18]. They speculate that this could be due to the effects of cannabis impairing neocortical areas that typically inhibit impulsivity, namely the prefrontal cortex, the anterior cingulate gyrus, nucleus accumbens, and the amygdala [18]. High-potency cannabis may exacerbate this effect.

While 36 states have legalized medical cannabis, Colorado (along with Washington) was first to permit its legal use for adults desiring its recreational effects in 2012 [19]. Other states have since followed. However, each state regulates cannabis differently. Legal access to cannabis ranges from highly restrictive permitting only a small number of plants cultivated specifically for an individual to treat a medical condition, to a robust recreational dispensary industry selling high-potency product, as is the case for those of us practicing in Colorado. We certainly perceived an uptick in cannabis use-related problems soon after its recreational availability, such as self-inflicted injuries. Others appreciated an increase in medical complications such as cyclical vomiting and children presenting to emergency departments after unintended ingestion [20]. While we firmly believed that Mr. C was not intentionally trying to end his life, his self-harm was quite severe. Fortunately, his wife was awake and able to call for help. His living in an urban area meant quick access to the emergency medical services and to a trauma center. However, had he died from his self-inflicted injuries, it is quite likely his death would have been classified as a suicide, regardless of his intent. It is possible that there have been deaths attributed to suicide that were instead severe and impulsive self-harm (without intent to die) while intoxicated with cannabis. Colorado suicide data suggests a possible relationship between cannabis and self-harm in those whose deaths were classified as suicide. Figure 13.1 shows data from the Colorado Department of Public Health and Environment violent death reporting system. The percentage of deaths by suicide from 2008 to 2018 who also had positive toxicology findings for cannabis are shown. There is a pronounced and steady increase in percentage positive for cannabis in suicides after Colorado legalized its recreational use in November 2012. Indeed, the average percentage of persons dying by suicide from 2008–2012 who were also positive for cannabis was 7.80%. Following recreational legalization and 5 years thereafter, the average was 18.83%. This is a meaningful and statistically significant increase when using an independent samples *t* test: $t(9) = -6.20$, $p < 0.001$. This finding is consistent with a 2020 study that wonders whether increased potency found in recreational cannabis is related to self-harm [21]. Their dataset is compelling, as they evaluated insurance claims for more than *75 million individuals*, noting that there was an association between cannabis use and self-harm in men 40 years and under in states that have legalized recreational use. No association was found in states that did not legalize recreational use.

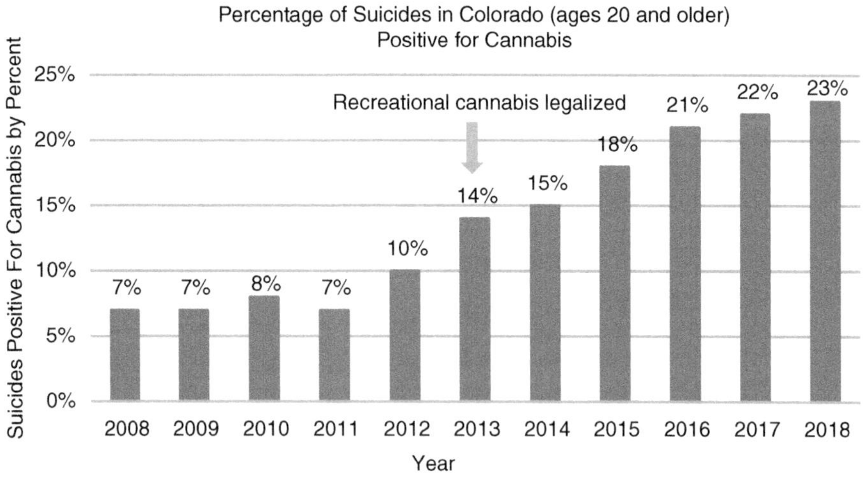

Fig. 13.1 Percentage of persons dying by suicide in Colorado who tested positive for cannabis by year, 2008 through 2018

Colorado kept its liquor stores and dispensaries open during the Covid-19 lockdown. With the "perfect storm" of physical distancing, economic downturn, and limited access to social opportunities, some researchers worry about increased suicide mortality [22]; the disturbing trend of increasing percentages of cannabis positive people among Colorado suicides is likely, unfortunately, to continue.

Treatment Approaches

Given the perception of cannabis as relatively safe, psychiatrists should counsel their patients about the dangers of its use. For some individuals it can provoke psychosis, depression, and anxiety. Indeed, for some patients, treating depression and anxiety may be complicated by ongoing cannabis use. Treatment plans should address cannabis use and caution given to patients that if they are seeking relief from many psychiatric conditions that they may have to abstain from cannabis.

When evaluating for risk of danger to self, there should be more attention paid to cannabis use. Infrequent use of a low potency product does not have the same risk as heavy (many times a week) use. High-potency cannabis is likely more dangerous and those who live in states that permit recreational sales should be aware of this. For some patients, part of their safety planning and means restriction may also need to address cannabis use for high-risk patients. Young men with frequent high potency use who have additional risk factors are at increased risk for suicide. A cautious approach to managing such individuals during times of crisis is encouraged.

Mr. C was evaluated almost daily during his 13-day hospital admission. His history and behavior before the incident was corroborated by his wife, other family members, and friends. He was consistently found to be euthymic, free from thoughts of self-harm, and appropriately concerned about the events that required hospital admission. There was no indication of psychiatric decompensation, acute stress disorder, nor modifiable risk factors for self-harm. He was warned that our team believed that intoxication of high-potency cannabis was the likely culprit and urged abstinence. He agreed with our conclusion and asked for outpatient resources for psychotherapy which we provided. Several weeks following his discharge he was readmitted for complications related to his surgical repair (infection and fluid collection). He has had no further contact with any of our behavioral health providers.

Summary

Numerous studies have sought to examine the relationship between cannabis use and self-harm. This is a complicated relationship with numerous moderating variables and confounds. This literature is almost exclusively correlational in nature and only a single study convincingly weighs in on cause and effect. Further, it is a heterogeneous literature comprising studies with large sample sizes (one cited earlier has an *n* of more than 75 million), meta-analyses, longitudinal data, and involves cannabis users from many different counties. Well-designed studies using similar methodologies have disparate findings. It is difficult to definitively answer the question whether risk of self-harm, including suicide, rises with cannabis use.

However, despite the heterogeneity of this literature, there are **compelling reasons** to conclude that cannabis use, particularly high potency forms of the drug, is associated with an increased risk of self-harm. As the clinical case from this chapter illustrates, had Mr. C simply refrained from high-potency cannabis the evening he stabbed himself, the odds that he would have engaged in self-harm are vanishingly small. The suicide data presented earlier from Colorado before and after the legalization of recreational cannabis is quite concerning. Not only are persons who have died by suicide positive for cannabis significantly higher after legalization, but the positivity rates have also steadily risen every year. There is no reason to believe—particularly with concern about the mental health effects of the Covid-19 pandemic—that this trend will change. Finally, it would be reassuring if the literature consistently showed no relationship between cannabis use and self-harm. It does not. There are convincing studies suggesting this relationship. Indeed, one study argues cogently for a cause-and-effect relationship between heavy cannabis use and self-harm in some men. At present, there is enough scholarship to raise an alarm that cannabis may be associated with self-harm. We should treat our patients with this in mind.

Highlights Box 13.1 Key Points for Patient Psychoeducation

- The literature examining the relationship between self-harm and cannabis use is almost entirely correlational in nature.
- It is a heterogeneous literature often with conflicting findings.
- Despite its heterogeneity, there are convincing studies finding an association between cannabis use and increased risk for self-harm.
- A single study finds a causal effect between heavy cannabis use and self-harm in men.
- The same study demonstrates that cannabis use does not increase with suicidal thoughts in men and women.
- In Colorado, deaths classified both as suicide and positive for cannabis nearly tripled following the legalization of recreational cannabis.
- Higher potency cannabis is associated with higher rates of self-harm.

Highlights Box 13.2 Key Points in Treatment and Management

- Despite Americans' perception that cannabis (particularly varieties that are sold legally) is safe, there is significant evidence showing some users may experience anxiety, psychosis, depression, and self-harm.
- This perception may lead some patients to not report their cannabis use to a global query about whether they use illicit substances.
- Psychiatrists and other mental health clinicians should also not work under this misperception; cannabis use may be associated with anxiety that is

refractory to treatment, a contributor to psychosis and depression, as well as self-harm (including suicide).
- When assessing those who endorse cannabis use, it is important to understand whether the patient is using a high or low potency substance, how frequent is the use, and whether onset of the signs and symptoms of mental illness is temporally related using the drug.
- Even for those who do not misuse cannabis, its users may still be at increased risk of self-harm.
- Safety assessments regarding risk for self-harm should routinely incorporate questions about cannabis use (beyond just whether substance misuse is part of the clinical case).
- Frequent and/or high-potency cannabis use, particularly in men, should raise the index of suspicion during safety evaluations.

References

1. Drapeau CW, McIntosh JL. U.S.A. suicide: 2019 official final data. Washington, DC: American Association of Suicidology; 2020. wwwsuicidologyorg. Acessed 1 March 2021.
2. Olfson M, Blanco C, Wall M, Liu S-M, Saha TD, Pickering RP, et al. National trends in suicide attempts among adults in the United States. JAMA Psychiat. 2017;74(11):1095–103.
3. Baldessarini RJ. Epidemiology of suicide: recent developments. Epidemiol Psychiatr Sci. 2020;29:e71. https://doi.org/10.1017/s2045796019000672.
4. Padmanathan P, Hall K, Moran P, Jones HE, Gunnell D, Carlisle V, et al. Prevention of suicide and reduction of self-harm among people with substance use disorder: a systematic review and meta-analysis of randomised controlled trials. Compr Psychiatry. 2020;96:152135. https://doi.org/10.1016/j.comppsych.2019.152135.
5. Ferrari AJ, Norman RE, Freedman G, Baxter AJ, Pirkis JE, Harris MG, et al. The burden attributable to mental and substance use disorders as risk factors for suicide: findings from the global burden of disease study 2010. PLoS One. 2014;9(4):e91936. https://doi.org/10.1371/journal.pone.0091936.
6. Carliner H, Brown QL, Sarvet AL, Hasin DS. Cannabis use, attitudes, and legal status in the U.S.: a review. Prev Med. 2017;104:13–23. https://doi.org/10.1016/j.ypmed.2017.07.008.
7. Fataar F, Goodman S, Wadsworth E, Hammond D. Consumer perceptions of 'legal' and 'illegal' cannabis in US states with legal cannabis sales. Addict Behav. 2021;112:106563. https://doi.org/10.1016/j.addbeh.2020.106563.
8. Kedzior KK, Laeber LT. A positive association between anxiety disorders and cannabis use or cannabis use disorders in the general population-a meta-analysis of 31 studies. BMC Psychiatry. 2014;14(1):1–22.
9. Gobbi G, Atkin T, Zytynski T, Wang S, Askari S, Boruff J, et al. Association of cannabis use in adolescence and risk of depression, anxiety, and suicidality in young adulthood: a systematic review and meta-analysis. JAMA Psychiat. 2019;76(4):426–34. https://doi.org/10.1001/jamapsychiatry.2018.4500.
10. Manrique-Garcia E, Zammit S, Dalman C, Hemmingsson T, Allebeck P. Cannabis use and depression: a longitudinal study of a national cohort of Swedish conscripts. BMC Psychiatry. 2012;12(1):112. https://doi.org/10.1186/1471-244X-12-112.
11. Price C, Hemmingsson T, Lewis G, Zammit S, Allebeck P. Cannabis and suicide: longitudinal study. Br J Psychiatry. 2009;195(6):492–7. https://doi.org/10.1192/bjp.bp.109.065227.

12. Pedersen W. Does cannabis use lead to depression and suicidal behaviours? A population-based longitudinal study. Acta Psychiatr Scand. 2008;118(5):395–403.
13. Borges G, Bagge CL, Orozco R. A literature review and meta-analyses of cannabis use and suicidality. J Affect Disord. 2016;195:63–74. https://doi.org/10.1016/j.jad.2016.02.007.
14. Beautrais AL, Joyce PR, Mulder RT. Cannabis abuse and serious suicide attempts. Addiction. 1999;94(8):1155–64. https://doi.org/10.1046/j.1360-0443.1999.94811555.x.
15. Van Ours JC, Williams J, Fergusson D, Horwood LJ. Cannabis use and suicidal ideation. J Health Econ. 2013;32(3):524–37.
16. Ahsaini M, Tazi F, Khalouk A, Lahlaidi K, Bouazzaoui A, Stuurman-Wieringa RE, et al. Bilateral testicular self-castration due to cannabis abuse: a case report. J Med Case Rep. 2011;5(1):1–4.
17. Delteil C, Sastre C, Piercecchi MD, Faget-Agius C, Deveaux M, Kintz P, et al. Death by self-mutilation after oral cannabis consumption. Leg Med (Tokyo). 2018;30:5–9. https://doi.org/10.1016/j.legalmed.2017.10.010.
18. Escelsior A, Murri MB, Corsini GP, Serafini G, Aguglia A, Zampogna D, et al. Cannabinoid use and self-injurious behaviours: a systematic review and meta-analysis. J Affect Disord. 2021;278:85.
19. Patton DV. A history of United States cannabis law. J Law Health. 2020;34(1):1–29.
20. Monte AA, Zane RD, Heard KJ. The implications of marijuana legalization in Colorado. JAMA. 2015;313(3):241–2. https://doi.org/10.1001/jama.2014.17057.
21. Matthay EC, Kiang MV, Elser H, Schmidt L, Humphreys K. Evaluation of State Cannabis Laws and Rates of self-harm and assault. JAMA Netw Open. 2021;4(3):e211955.
22. Reger MA, Stanley IH, Joiner TE. Suicide mortality and coronavirus disease 2019-a perfect storm? JAMA Psychiat. 2020;77(11):1093–4. https://doi.org/10.1001/jamapsychiatry.2020.1060.

Cannabis in the Adult Medical and Consultation-Liaison Settings

14

Heather Murray and Thida Thant

Complications of Cannabis Use in the Medical Setting

Case

Mr. Deer is a 66-year-old man with history of remote cerebrovascular accident admitted to the internal medicine service for altered mental status. Due to his confusion, it is difficult to obtain a detailed history, but collateral information reveals he uses cannabis daily for chronic nausea and vomiting with progressive increase in potency over the last year. Prior medical hospitalizations were for dehydration, vomiting, and altered mental status and he has been noted to become increasingly irritable over the course of hospital stays and at times asks to leave again medical advice. During this admission, physical and mental status exam are remarkable for increased rigidity of bilateral upper extremities, mutism, poor attention, and echolalia, and he is intermittently agitated and restless with dysregulated sleep. Complete metabolic panel and complete blood count are unremarkable, though urine drug screen is positive for cannabinoids and head imaging is notable for chronic microvascular changes and evidence of former stroke. The primary medical team is concerned that his mental status is not improving despite several days in the hospital and no clear underlying etiology.

Introduction and Literature Review

This case will be remarkably familiar to the consultation-liaison (C-L) psychiatrist. Patients are frequently admitted for delirium of unclear etiology with multiple complicating factors such as age, prior medical conditions, and substance use. With the

H. Murray (✉) · T. Thant
Department of Psychiatry, University of Colorado School of Medicine, Aurora, CO, USA
e-mail: heather.j.murray@cuanschutz.edu; Thida.thant@cuanschutz.edu

P. Riggs, T. Thant (eds.), *Cannabis in Psychiatric Practice*, Psychiatry Update 3,
https://doi.org/10.1007/978-3-031-04874-6_14

increasing prevalence of cannabis legalization and medicalization over the years, more and more patients present to medical settings with both recreational and medical cannabis use. However, history of cannabis use is often overlooked in favor of searching for more acute medical issues and more traditionally dangerous substances such as illicit stimulants and opioids. But what is the relevance of cannabis use and how often should we consider cannabis use within our differential diagnosis of a patient presenting similarly? In the above case there are multiple concerns: altered mental status, history of possibly high-potency cannabis use, chronic nausea and vomiting, history of prior stroke, history of depression, and signs of catatonia. Where to begin?

Delirium

Cannabis use and withdrawal are frequently overlooked as contributing factors to delirium. Per DSM-5 [1] criteria, delirium is defined as a waxing and waning disturbance in level of awareness and reduced ability to focus, sustain, and shift attention that develops over hours to days and is a clear change from baseline mental status. Delirium can be accompanied by disturbance in sleep/wake cycle, perceptual disturbances, affective and mood disturbances, delusional thought content, and psychomotor disturbances [2, 3].

Delirium evaluation should include a general medical workup, detailed history (including collateral information), and thorough physical exam to uncover etiology of the patient's presentation. In Mr. Deer's case, collateral and urine drug screen would have been particularly helpful to identify history of heavy cannabis use.

Literature review of delirium associated with cannabis use and withdrawal is limited to several case studies. In one case study, an 82-year-old woman unintentionally ingested several cannabis laden cookies at her daughter's home leading to a short course of delirium requiring medical hospitalization [4]. In a second case study, a 49-year-old man developed 1–2 days of altered mental status 13 days into his medical admission and was found to have consumed cannabis laced baked goods in his hospital room [5]. In a third case study, a 71-year-old woman became delirious due to presumed dronabinol withdrawal that improved with restarting the medication [6].

The above case studies reveal the importance of obtaining collateral and maintaining an index of suspicion for cannabis use as a cause for delirium, even for patients with no history of cannabis use, medicinal cannabis use, or with new onset delirium days to weeks into hospitalization. All the patients avoided invasive, costly, and potential harmful medical workup because of judicious history gathering.

How might cannabis cause delirium? THC-related psychiatric symptoms appear to stem from its interaction with CB1 receptors in the central nervous system [4]. As discussed in previous chapters, potency of THC in recreational cannabis strains has increased substantially since legalization in many states [7]. In addition, growers and dispensaries continue to alter the makeup of the cannabis plant leading to lower concentrations of CBD, which is protective against the negative psychoactive effects of THC including anxiety and psychosis [6]. As legalization of recreational cannabis becomes more common throughout the world, the ratio of THC:CBD will continue to grow in medicinal and recreational strains leading to higher risk of development of delirium associated with cannabis use.

In addition to direct effects on the CNS, the astute C-L psychiatrist should consider that THC inhibits the cytochrome P450 enzyme CYP2C9, which causes increased serum concentrations of this enzyme's pharmacological substrates. These substrates include medications with narrow therapeutic windows, such as warfarin [8], and several centrally acting medications. When considering medication dose changes, initiation of new medications, or workup of delirium secondary to polypharmacy, one should screen for chronic cannabis use as it may affect metabolism of other drugs for weeks to months due to its lipophilicity [9].

Catatonia

Another consideration in this case is catatonia due to findings of mutism, echolalia, and upper extremity rigidity. Catatonia is a neuropsychiatric syndrome characterized by signs of withdrawal, abnormal movements, and abnormal behaviors including stupor, catalepsy, waxy flexibility, mutism, negativism, posturing, mannerisms, stereotypy, agitation, echolalia, and echopraxia [1]. While traditionally described as a schizophrenia subtype, in some studies, catatonia secondary to a medical condition accounted for upwards of half of presenting cases [10], demonstrating the need for thorough history and medical evaluation in patients with signs of catatonia, particularly in those without a psychiatric history.

Catatonia associated with cannabis use and withdrawal is only described in case studies, but it appears to be consistent with classical presentation and responds well to traditional treatments including lorazepam. One case study describes a young woman in her twenties with no significant psychiatry history admitted to psychiatry for new onset mood symptoms and catatonia that improved with lorazepam treatment [11]. The second case describes another young woman with schizophrenia history admitted to the hospital for failure to thrive and disorganized behaviors. She endorsed using high-potency cannabis daily, was diagnosed with catatonia, and signs and symptoms resolved with treatment with lorazepam and home antipsychotic [11]. A third case study discusses a young man with known history of periodic catatonia in context of heavy cannabis use admitted for new episode of catatonia after he recently increased his cannabis use [12]. A fourth case study describes a young man with intellectual disability and heavy cannabis use, but no other psychiatric history, who developed catatonia while incarcerated due to cannabis withdrawal. He made a full recovery with lorazepam and abstinence from cannabis [13]. The final case describes a young man with history of long-term heavy cannabis use admitted for treatment of psychosis and catatonia who showed robust response to lorazepam treatment with no additional catatonic episodes with abstinence from cannabis [14].

How might cannabis increase risk for catatonia? Animal studies have shown that chronic THC use can decrease extracellular glutamate and increase GABA levels in the brain [13]. Abrupt cessation of cannabis may disrupt this glutamate/GABA balance causing D2 receptor hypoactivity which could lead to catatonia [13]. Notably, synthetic cannabinoids, which are full CB1 and CB2 agonists that bind to the receptors with much higher affinity than THC, have also been associated with psychosis and catatonia in several case studies. Their use is also associated with high rates of other psychiatric symptoms including delirium, anxiety, and psychosis. Given the changing ratios and concentrations of CBD and THC in modern cannabis strains, there is question of whether these new strains more reflect receptor activity of synthetic cannabinoids than traditional cannabis strains, which in turn would explain increasing presentation of catatonia associated with high-potency cannabis strains.

Cannabis Hyperemesis Syndrome

Though not yet an acute concern in Mr. Deer's case, his history of escalating cannabis use and ongoing nausea and vomiting outside the hospital places him at risk for development of cannabis hyperemesis syndrome. First described in 2004 by Allen et al. [15], cannabinoid hyperemesis syndrome (CHS) is defined as a syndrome of cyclical vomiting related to chronic, high-dose cannabis use that is often associated with compulsive engagement in hot baths and showers to control symptoms. CHS consists of three phrases, which are described in Table 14.1.

The actual prevalence of CHS is unknown but the syndrome is believed to be underdiagnosed. Patients often present to the emergency department with intractable nausea and vomiting over the course of a day to a little over a week. The differential for these symptoms is quite broad, including medical emergencies, so patients are at risk for expensive workup, iatrogenic harm, and significant delays in diagnosis [15]. Cyclic vomiting syndrome (CVS) is a functional GI disorder that must be differentiated from CHS with the key difference being temporality of symptoms. CVS patients often have gastrointestinal symptoms that predate initiation or increase in cannabis use, while CHS patients have heavy cannabis use predating their symptoms [17]. In 92.3% of CHS cases, symptoms improved with hot baths and showers, and in most cases, symptoms resolved completely with cessation from cannabis [18].

The endocannabinoid system is involved in GI motility [19], appetite, and nausea [20]. The leading theory explaining the relationship between cannabis use and CHS is that heavy cannabis use causes dysregulation of the endocannabinoid system of the brain and gastrointestinal tract. THC binds to CB1 receptors in the GI tract leading to decreased GI motility and gastric emptying which may then contribute to

Table 14.1 Cannabinoid hyperemesis syndrome criteria and phases [13, 14]

Prodromal phase	Nausea, anorexia, and abdominal pain lasting months to years
Hyperemesis phase	Cyclical vomiting, severe nausea, abdominal pain and relief with hot baths/showers lasting 1–10 days
Postdrome phase	Recovery with progressive improvement in symptoms over weeks to months after cessation of cannabis
Rome IV Criteria [16]	Symptoms must be present for the past 3 months, symptomatic onset occurring at least 6 months prior to diagnosis, stereotypical episodes lasting <1 week, at least three episodes within the past year and no vomiting between episodes

hyperemesis [21]. In addition to the above, THC displays a biphasic effect, it may dysregulate stress responses, and it causes vasculature dilation and autonomic dysfunction that are beyond the scope of this chapter.

Cannabis Withdrawal

A final consideration in Mr. Deer's case is cannabis withdrawal, a clinical syndrome frequently overlooked as it often lacks the same acuity and medical risk as other withdrawal syndromes. While difficult to assess in Mr. Deer given his altered mental status, possible signs of withdrawal include restlessness, agitation, and sleep disruption. Cannabis withdrawal first appeared as a psychiatric diagnosis in the DSM-5 and is characterized by irritability, aggression, anxiety, sleep difficulty, decreased appetite/weight loss, restlessness, and depressed mood within 1 week of abrupt cessation or reduction in cannabis use plus physical symptoms of abdominal pain, tremors, sweating, fever, chills, and headache. It occurs in 12.1% of frequent cannabis users with risk factors including diagnosis of mood disorder, anxiety disorder, personality disorder, or family history of depression but no personal or family history of other substance use disorders [22]. Symptoms often begin within 24 h of cessation, peak within 1 week, and last up to 1 month [23]. As rates of cannabis use increase, it is key the C-L psychiatrist consider withdrawal as a potential source for different psychiatric symptoms including delirium, catatonia, insomnia, anxiety, and agitation. Though not thought to be life-threatening, cannabis withdrawal can be uncomfortable, and for patients accustomed to using cannabis for a variety of symptoms, it can be a difficult experience to undergo "forced" abstinence while in the hospital and may contribute to discharge against medical advice.

Treatment Approaches

Now that you can identify syndromes related to cannabis use in the consultation-liaison psychiatry setting, what are the approaches to treatment? As discussed above, history and collateral information are key, though in many of these cases it is impossible to do the kind of evaluation discussed earlier in this text until the patient's mental status improves. While it may be tempting to move on once the patient improves, the opportunity for psychoeducation is lost if cannabis use is not addressed prior to discharge from the hospital.

Delirium

The literature related to management of cannabis induced delirium is relatively limited. One case series [24] discussed treatment of agitated delirium presumed to be related to cannabis withdrawal in three young adults. In all three cases, the agitation was resistant to traditional management, including antipsychotics, but responded quickly to dexmedetomidine. Dexmedetomidine is a highly selective alpha-2 agonist used to manage agitated delirium in the ICU [25]. Its short half-life and transient side effects of hypotension and bradycardia make it an excellent option to manage symptoms of agitated delirium [24]. In Mr. Deer's case, if there was a lower suspicion for catatonia and his agitation were to worsen, dexmedetomidine would be key to consider before further escalation of antipsychotics or use of additional sedative-hypnotics such as benzodiazepines.

Catatonia

Though differentiating between "organic" catatonia and delirium can be difficult in the acute medical setting, the cases described above indicate that cannabis induced catatonia responds to conventional treatments of catatonia, primarily lorazepam, with the added importance of abstinence from cannabis to minimize chance of recurrence [11–14]. In Mr. Deer's case, the lack of improvement in mental status over several days combined with echolalia, mutism, and rigidity warrant a lorazepam challenge to rule out the possibility of catatonia [26].

Cannabis Hyperemesis Syndrome

Though low on the list of priorities in Mr. Deer's case at this time, discussion of his risk for development of CHS will be a key part of his psychoeducation prior to discharge from the hospital. By far the most definitive treatment for CHS is abstinence from cannabis [18]. However, abstinence takes weeks to months to have an effect, so patients often require acute symptomatic treatment of the hyperemesis phase. CHS patients may be hospitalized for dehydration and acute kidney injury, so fluid resuscitation, antiemetics, and electrolyte replacement are cornerstones of management [27]. There are several case studies that discuss subjective success of dopamine antagonists, such as haloperidol, which may counteract the increased dopamine synthesis THC perpetuates [28] with some studies showing an 81% response of CHS symptoms in patients receiving 1–5 mg of haloperidol for acute nausea and vomiting [29]. Droperidol has also been found helpful in a case series; however, use of this medication is limited within the USA due to its black box warning for prolonged QTc [30]. It is important to obtain an EKG and electrolyte levels if recommending haloperidol or droperidol for CHS given the high frequency of electrolyte abnormalities found in these patients. Multiple case studies and series have shown at least partial response of symptoms in patients treated with topical capsaicin cream applied to the abdomen [31–34] and its use is associated with lower use of opioids and less time in the emergency department [35]. Capsaicin is theorized to normalize the TRVP-1 receptor activity (similar to heat from hot showers and baths) leading to transient improvement in nausea and vomiting [36]. Conventional antiemetics have demonstrated poor effect [28] while opioids are known to worsen gastric immobility [36]. While there is evidence for the antiemetic effects of benzodiazepines via GABA receptors in the GI tract, their use should be minimized in chronic treatment of CHS as these patients often meet criteria for use disorders [28]. A retrospective review of dronabinol in the emergency department found length of stay and use of other antiemetics were reduced in patients given dronabinol versus those provided standard of care [30]. However, given the theorized mechanisms underlying CHS one would question whether treatment with CB1 agonists would simply the onset of or even worsen CHS symptoms.

Table 14.2 Pharmacological treatment of cannabis withdrawal

Medication	Targeted symptoms	Dosing if available
May be helpful for specific symptoms of withdrawal		
Mirtazapine [37]	Sleep and appetite	Up to 30 mg nightly
Zolpidem [38]	Sleep	12.5 mg QHS ER
Gabapentin [39]	Cravings, withdrawal, and executive functioning	Titrated up to 300 mg BID and 600 mg qPM in clinical trials
Guanfacine [40]	Irritability, sleep	2 mg QHS
Dronabinol [41]	Cravings, appetite, mood, tension	30–90 mg/day in divided doses
Nabiximols [42]	Irritability, depression, cravings, insomnia, anxiety, appetite, restlessness	8 sprays QID
Quetiapine [43]	Appetite, insomnia	200 mg/day in divided doses
Not found to be helpful		
Bupropion [44]		
Venlafaxine [45]		
Depakote [46]		
Lithium [47]		

Cannabis Withdrawal

Each day Mr. Deer remains in the hospital, his risk of withdrawal from cannabis increases, especially given his escalating use prior to admission. Table 14.2 below summarizes the current evidence regarding pharmacological treatment of cannabis withdrawal symptoms. It should be noted that many of these studies are small, proof of concept studies with high dropout rates and a heterogeneity of patient populations. However, most of these medications are quite safe and their use may lead to a more comfortable medical hospitalization.

Conclusion

Though historically viewed as much safer than other substances such as alcohol, stimulants, or opiates, cannabis use is not benign and may contribute to acute medical issues including delirium, catatonia, intractable vomiting, and withdrawal. Cannabis can impact clinical presentations in acute medical settings in a variety of ways and it is increasingly important for C-L psychiatrists to be aware of these effects.

Once a diagnosis and etiology are determined, the C-L psychiatrist must consider the importance of their role regarding psychoeducation. If a patient's altered mental status or catatonia is thought possibly related to cannabis, education is key to decrease risk for repeated hospitalizations. For accidental ingestions or overdose, psychoeducation about safe storage and labeling may be more important. For patients experiencing CHS or cannabis withdrawal, these discussions may be challenging as patients often feel that cannabis is helpful for symptoms they are experiencing and may struggle to tolerate the withdrawal period without additional support. Highlights Box 14.1 includes highlights from this chapter to share with patients.

As discussed throughout this chapter, while the literature may be sparse, it is compelling and especially worth considering in our more confusing or refractory cases of altered mental status. As rates of use increase in our country and cannabis becomes less stigmatized, cannabis should be considered in any patient presenting with altered mental status or agitation, particularly the elderly and in cases of new onset delirium days to weeks into a hospitalization. In addition to recreational cannabis use, the prescribed use of pharmaceutical cannabinoids such as dronabinol or nabiximols carry some of the same risks of intoxication and withdrawal as their THC analogs. Highlights Box 14.2 summarizes key takeaway considerations in treatment and management of cannabis related delirium, catatonia, hyperemesis syndrome, and withdrawal.

Highlights Box 14.1 Key Points for Patient Psychoeducation

- Cannabis withdrawal is a new diagnosis found in the DSM-5 and is characterized by signs and symptoms that begin within 1 week of abrupt cessation or reduction in cannabis use.
- Consider cannabis intoxication and withdrawal in all cases of delirium, even in elderly patients, those without a use history, and patients with a prolonged hospital stay.
- With increased use of THC analogs for medicinal reasons, maintain an index of suspicion for possible contribution to delirium in patients who are prescribed these analogs.
- Changes in THC:CBD ratio likely leads to increased risk of psychiatric side effects of modern recreational and medicinal cannabis strains including delirium.
- The literature examining association of cannabis use with catatonia is limited, but with increasing ratio of THC:CBD in recreational and medicinal strains, the prevalence of medical complications from cannabis use will likely increase.

Highlights Box 14.2 Key Points in Treatment and Management

- Dexmedetomidine appears to be safe and efficacious for treatment of agitated delirium associated with cannabis intoxication and withdrawal.
- Catatonia associated with cannabis use and withdrawal appears to respond to standard treatments including lorazepam.
- The best treatment for CHS is abstinence from cannabis but improvement can take weeks to months.
- Evidence of pharmacological treatment in CHS is limited, but first-line medications include haloperidol, droperidol, and topical capsaicin cream to the abdomen. Benzodiazepines are also likely helpful, but use is limited

given addiction potential. THC analogs may help in the short term but have the potential to delay or worsen CHS symptoms.
- Mirtazapine, quetiapine, and guanfacine may treat specific symptoms of cannabis withdrawal, but do not reduce risk of relapse or improve cravings.
- Zolpidem may assist in management of sleep disturbances but do not improve risk for relapse or cravings.
- CB1 agonists like THC and nabiximols may help treat most withdrawal symptoms and may even reduce risk of relapse.

References

1. American Psychiatric Association: diagnostic and statistical manual of mental disorders, 5th edition. Arlington: American Psychiatric Association; 2013.
2. Franco JG, Trzepacz PT, Meagher DJ, Kean J, Lee Y, Kim J-L, et al. Three core domains of delirium validated using exploratory and confirmatory factor analyses. Psychosomatics. 2013;54(3):227–38.
3. Wilner A. Cookie encephalopathy. Medscape Psychiatry; 2013. https://www.medscape.com/viewarticle/807778_1 Accessed June, 2021.
4. Fine C, Kishel B, O'Glasser AY, Desai SS. A greener oregon: acute inpatient delirium. Am J Med. 2017;130(4):423–5.
5. Muramatsu RS, Silva N, Ahmed I. Suspected dronabinol withdrawal in an elderly cannabis-naive medically ill patient. Am J Psychiatry. 2013;170(7):804.
6. ElSohly MA, Mehmedic Z, Foster S, Gon C, Chandra S, Church JC. Changes in cannabis potency over the last 2 decades (1995-2014): analysis of current data in the United States. Biol Psychiatry. 2016;79(7):613–9.
7. Greger J, Bates V, Mechtler L, Gengo F. A review of cannabis and interactions with anticoagulant and antiplatelet agents. J Clin Pharmacol. 2020;60(4):432–8.
8. Citti C, Braghiroli D, Vandelli MA, Cannazza G. Pharmaceutical and biomedical analysis of cannabinoids: a critical review. J Pharm Biomed Anal. 2018;147:565–79.
9. Denysenko L, Sica N, Penders TM, Philbrick KL, Walker A, Shaffer S, et al. Catatonia in the medically ill: etiology, diagnosis, and treatment. The Academy of Consultation-Liaison Psychiatry Evidence-Based Medicine Subcommittee Monograph. Ann Clin Psychiatry. 2018;30(2):140–55.
10. Mekala H, Malik Z, Lone J, Shah K, Ishaq M. Cannabis-induced catatonia: a case series. Cureus. 2020;12(6):e8603.
11. Bajaj B, Pathak P, Mehrotra S, Singh V, Govil S, Khanna A. Cannabis induced periodic catatonia: a case report. Int J Ment Health Addict. 2011;9:162–4.
12. Caudron M, Rolland B, Deheul S, Geoffroy PA, Thomas P, Amad A. Catatonia and cannabis withdrawal: a case report. Subst Abus. 2016;37(1):188–9.
13. Manning T, Bartow C, McNaughton M, Reynolds E, Chen Z. Vaping cannabis oil: a case of catatonia associated with use of high-potency cannabis. Psychosomatics. 2020;61(6): 745–51.
14. Allen JH, de Moore GM, Heddle R, Twartz JC. Cannabinoid hyperemesis: cyclical hyperemesis in association with chronic cannabis abuse. Gut. 2004;53(11):1566–70.
15. Schmulson MJ, Drossman DA. What is new in Rome iv. J Neurogastroenterol Motil. 2017;23(2):151–63.
16. Perrotta G, Miller J, Stevens T, et al. Cannabinoid hyperemesis: relevance to emergency medicine. Acad Emerg Med. 2012;19:S286–S7.

17. Darmani NA. Cannabinoid-induced hyperemesis: a conundrum-from clinical recognition to basic science mechanisms. Pharmaceuticals (Basel). 2010;3(7):2163–77.
18. Sorensen CJ, DeSanto K, Borgelt L, Phillips KT, Monte AA. Cannabinoid hyperemesis syndrome: diagnosis, pathophysiology, and treatment-a systematic review. J Med Toxicol. 2017;13(1):71–87.
19. Izzo AA, Mascolo N, Pinto L, Capasso R, Capasso F. The role of cannabinoid receptors in intestinal motility, defaecation and diarrhoea in rats. Eur J Pharmacol. 1999;384(1):37–42.
20. Sharkey KA, Darmani NA, Parker LA. Regulation of nausea and vomiting by cannabinoids and the endocannabinoid system. Eur J Pharmacol. 2014;722:134–46.
21. Rock EM, Goodwin JM, Limebeer CL, Breuer A, Pertwee RG, Mechoulam R, et al. Interaction between non-psychotropic cannabinoids in marihuana: effect of cannabigerol (Cbg) on the anti-nausea or anti-emetic effects of cannabidiol (Cbd) in rats and shrews. Psychopharmacology. 2011;215(3):505–12.
22. Livne O, Shmulewitz D, Lev-Ran S, Hasin DS. DSM-5 cannabis withdrawal syndrome: demographic and clinical correlates in U.S. adults. Drug Alcohol Depend. 2019;195:170–7.
23. Bonnet U, Preuss UW. The cannabis withdrawal syndrome: current insights. Subst Abus Rehabil. 2017;8:9–37.
24. Leikin JB, Amusina O. Use of dexmedetomidine to treat delirium primarily caused by cannabis. Am J Emerg Med. 2017;35(3):524.e1–2.
25. Afonso J, Reis F. Dexmedetomidine: current role in anesthesia and intensive care. Rev Bras Anestesiol. 2012;62(1):118–33.
26. Sienaert P, Dhossche DM, Vancampfort D, De Hert M, Gazdag G. A clinical review of the treatment of catatonia. Front Psych. 2014;5:181.
27. Habboushe J, Sedor J. Cannabinoid hyperemesis acute renal failure: a common sequela of cannabinoid hyperemesis syndrome. Am J Emerg Med. 2014;32(6):690.e1–2.
28. Richards JR. Cannabinoid hyperemesis syndrome: a disorder of the HPA axis and sympathetic nervous system? Med Hypotheses. 2017;103:90–5.
29. Kast KA, Gershengoren L. Cannabinoid hyperemesis syndrome and the consulting psychiatrist: a case study of diagnosis and treatment for an emerging disorder in psychiatric practice. J Psychiatr Pract. 2018;24(1):51–5.
30. Lee C, Greene SL, Wong A. The utility of droperidol in the treatment of cannabinoid hyperemesis syndrome. Clin Toxicol (Phila). 2019;57(9):773–7.
31. Dezieck L, Hafez Z, Conicella A, Blohm E, O'Connor MJ, Schwarz ES, et al. Resolution of cannabis hyperemesis syndrome with topical capsaicin in the emergency department: a case series. Clin Toxicol (Phila). 2017;55(8):908–13.
32. Biary R, Oh A, Lapoint J, Nelson L, Hoffman R, Howland M. Topical capsaicin cream used as a therapy for cannabinoid hyperemesis syndrome. Clin Toxicol. 2014;52(7):787.
33. Lapoint J. Case series of patients treated for cannabinoid hyper-emesis syndrome with capsaicin cream. Annual meeting of the north American congress of clinical toxicology (NACCT). Clin Toxicol. 2014;52(7):707.
34. Román F, Llorens P, Burillo-Putze G. [Topical capsaicin cream in the treatment for cannabinoid hyperemesis syndrome]. Med Clin (Barc). 2016;147(11):517–8.
35. Wagner S, Hoppe J, Zuckerman M, Schwarz K, McLaughlin J. Efficacy and safety of topical capsaicin for cannabinoid hyperemesis syndrome in the emergency department. Clin Toxicol (Phila). 2020;58(6):471–5.
36. Yang F, Zheng J. Understand spiciness: mechanism of TRPV1 channel activation by capsaicin. Protein Cell. 2017;8(3):169–77.
37. Haney M, Hart CL, Vosburg SK, Comer SD, Reed SC, Cooper ZD, et al. Effects of baclofen and mirtazapine on a laboratory model of marijuana withdrawal and relapse. Psychopharmacology. 2010;211(2):233–44.
38. Brezing CA, Levin FR. The current state of pharmacological treatments for cannabis use disorder and withdrawal. Neuropsychopharmacology. 2018;43(1):173–94.

39. Mason BJ, Crean R, Goodell V, Light JM, Quello S, Shadan F, et al. A proof-of-concept randomized controlled study of gabapentin: effects on cannabis use, withdrawal and executive function deficits in cannabis-dependent adults. Neuropsychopharmacology. 2012;37(7):1689–98.
40. Haney M, Cooper ZD, Bedi G, Herrmann E, Comer SD, Reed SC, et al. Guanfacine decreases symptoms of cannabis withdrawal in daily cannabis smokers. Addict Biol. 2019;24(4):707–16.
41. Budney AJ, Vandrey RG, Hughes JR, Moore BA, Bahrenburg B. Oral delta-9-tetrahydrocannabinol suppresses cannabis withdrawal symptoms. Drug Alcohol Depend. 2007;86(1):22–9.
42. Allsop DJ, Copeland J, Lintzeris N, Dunlop AJ, Montebello M, Sadler C, et al. Nabiximols as an agonist replacement therapy during cannabis withdrawal: a randomized clinical trial. JAMA Psychiat. 2014;71(3):281–91.
43. Cooper ZD, Foltin RW, Hart CL, Vosburg SK, Comer SD, Haney M. A human laboratory study investigating the effects of quetiapine on marijuana withdrawal and relapse in daily marijuana smokers. Addict Biol. 2013;18(6):993–1002.
44. Haney M, Ward AS, Comer SD, Hart CL, Foltin RW, Fischman MW. Bupropion SR worsens mood during marijuana withdrawal in humans. Psychopharmacology. 2001;155(2):171–9.
45. Levin FR, Mariani J, Brooks DJ, Pavlicova M, Nunes EV, Agosti V, et al. A randomized double-blind, placebo-controlled trial of venlafaxine-extended release for co-occurring cannabis dependence and depressive disorders. Addiction. 2013;108(6):1084–94.
46. Haney M, Hart CL, Vosburg SK, Nasser J, Bennett A, Zubaran C, et al. Marijuana withdrawal in humans: effects of oral THC or divalproex. Neuropsychopharmacology. 2004;29(1):158–70.
47. Johnston J, Lintzeris N, Allsop DJ, Suraev A, Booth J, Carson DS, et al. Lithium carbonate in the management of cannabis withdrawal: a randomized placebo-controlled trial in an inpatient setting. Psychopharmacology. 2014;231(24):4623–36.

Cannabis in the Perinatal Period

15

Sarah Nagle-Yang and Parvaneh Nouri

Clinical Case

Andrea is a 23-year-old primigravid patient at 20 weeks gestation referred for a psychiatric evaluation by her OB/GYN after she scored an 18 on the Edinburgh Postnatal Depression Scale (EPDS) screening at her last prenatal care visit. She scored highest for the inventories of sad mood, excessive guilt, tearfulness, and reduced pleasure. She also endorsed poor sleep but attributes that to her pregnancy. Most concerning however, was her endorsement of sometimes having thoughts of harming herself. She denies active suicidal ideation, plan, or intent and does appear to have strong future-orientation as she mentions planning for baby's arrival. She states these passive suicidal thoughts have been harder to quell recently and as a way to cope she has resumed smoking cannabis a few times a week.

Introduction

Cannabis is the most widely used federally illicit substance in the United States [1]. It is reported that at least 1 in 5 adults between the ages of 18 and 25 endorse using cannabis within the past month [2]. Further, it is the most widely used recreational substance of abuse during pregnancy [3]. In the USA, as the landscape of state-based legislation has shifted toward legalization of both medical and recreational cannabis, its use has increased in the general population as well as among pregnant individuals. While legalization may confer improved regulation of production quality and sale, the concentration of the primary psychoactive cannabinoid tetrahydrocannabinol (THC) has increased 3–5 fold in commercial cannabis products in

S. Nagle-Yang (✉) · P. Nouri
Department of Psychiatry, University of Colorado Anschutz, Denver, CO, USA
e-mail: Sarah.nagle-yang@cuanschutz.edu; Parvaneh.nouri@cuanschutz.edu

P. Riggs, T. Thant (eds.), *Cannabis in Psychiatric Practice*, Psychiatry Update 3,
https://doi.org/10.1007/978-3-031-04874-6_15

Europe and North America, from approximately 3% to 10–15% between 2008 and 2016 and the variety of products available and subsequent mode(s) of consumption vastly differ from decades past [4]. The commercialization of cannabis and its rapidly diversifying market has superseded the pace of research, particularly within the realm of reproductive safety. Now, more than ever, it is imperative to understand the impact of cannabis on mental health and behavior as well as its safety during pregnancy and lactation.

While there continues to be a paucity of literature describing the effects of cannabis use during pregnancy and during lactation, the body of knowledge is growing. Existing data suggest that cannabis use during pregnancy may have implications on obstetrical outcomes and fetal development, that THC is excreted into breastmilk and metabolized by breastfed infants, and that secondhand cannabis smoke may be associated with sudden infant death syndrome (SIDS). Emerging epidemiologic data also describe risk factors for use during pregnancy and commonly reported reasons for use during pregnancy. A more nuanced understanding of cannabis use during pregnancy and lactation may allow for a more effective and sensitive approach by providers.

This chapter serves to inform psychiatric and obstetrical providers on the topic of cannabis use during the perinatal period. While variability exists on how the "perinatal period" is defined, for the purposes of this chapter we will consider the perinatal period to include the full gestational period until 1 year postpartum. In this chapter we discuss the epidemiology of cannabis use during pregnancy, risk factors that may predispose one to use during pregnancy, reported reasons for use, and clinical recommendations for approaching the patient using cannabis during pregnancy. The authors of this chapter seek to impart guidance for care based on the principles of trauma-informed care and harm reduction. Additional considerations regarding pharmacokinetics of cannabis use during lactation period will be discussed. While brief references to data regarding cannabis use and fetal development may be made in this chapter, the reader can reference Chap. 3 for a complete discussion of that topic.

A Note on CBD

Historically, literature regarding cannabis use has focused on the psychoactive cannabinoid, THC. However, apart from THC there are numerous other phytocannabinoids identified in cannabis, including a more recent cannabinoid of focus, cannabidiol (CBD). There exists a growing commercial market for products that contain CBD either in conjunction with THC or even by itself. However, for the purposes of concision and given that most of the data regarding reproductive safety currently focuses solely on THC, this chapter will not focus on CBD (refer to Chap. 3 for further details on CBD). Further investigation and discussion on the pharmacokinetic properties of CBD during pregnancy are warranted.

Clinical Case

Upon clinical interview, you learn more about Andrea's social history. You find that she is single/never married and denies involvement of the partner with whom she became pregnant. Andrea lives in a one-bedroom apartment though states she is considering moving in with a friend out of financial concern. She only recently obtained medical insurance for the first time in her adult life, after enrolling in Medicaid for prenatal care. Further discussion reveals that while she wants to continue her pregnancy, the pregnancy was unintended.

- *How do these factors impact her risk for cannabis use, particularly during pregnancy?*
- *What are the most common reasons cited for cannabis use during pregnancy?*
- *How do these factors impact and guide clinical practice?*

Epidemiology and Risk Factors

As states legalize cannabis for both medical and recreational sale, the prevalence of cannabis use in the United States has increased in both the general population and perinatal individuals. The National Survey on Drug Use and Health (NSDUH) suggests that use in the general population more than doubled between 2002 and 2014 and use during pregnancy rose nearly 65% during that period [5]. Substance Abuse and Mental Health Services (SAMHSA) survey data estimates use during pregnancy in the United States has increased from 3.4% in 2015 to 4.7% in 2018 [2]. These values may be an underestimation of true rates of use during pregnancy as these data are collected by survey and self-reports while cannabis is still not federally legal and its use during pregnancy is stigmatized and largely not recommended by professional collectives in healthcare.

Pregnant persons who reported cannabis use within the last 30 days were three times as likely to fall into the age category of 18–25 years than the age category of 25–44 years, suggesting generational differences in cannabis use during pregnancy (Brown et al. 2017). Another interpretation of these data may be that younger individuals are at increased risk for using cannabis during pregnancy.

The Pregnancy Risk Assessment Monitoring System (cleverly referred to as PRAMS) was developed in 1987 by the Centers for Disease Control and Prevention (CDC) and has since been adopted by state health departments. A recent analysis of aggregate data from eight states' PRAMS surveys (Alaska, Illinois, Maine, New Mexico, New York, North Dakota, Pennsylvania, and West Virginia) found that those who reported use of cannabis during pregnancy were more likely to identify themselves as unmarried, <25 years old, and with 12 years of education or less (Ko et al. 2020). PRAMS respondents reporting cannabis use during pregnancy were also more likely to report concurrent tobacco use relative to respondents who did not report cannabis use [6].

Another analysis of PRAMS data from Alaska, Colorado, Maine, Michigan, and Washington found relationships between perinatal cannabis use and several "Stressful Life Events (SLEs)." Examples of SLEs include divorce/loss of relationship, losing income source/job or partner losing their job, difficulty paying rent and other essential costs of living, partner not desiring the pregnancy, incarceration or partner's incarceration, and close association with others who use substances. Of the SLEs surveyed amongst respondents who had delivered an infant within the last 6 months, three SLEs were significantly associated with cannabis use during pregnancy and one was associated with cannabis use in the postpartum period. These SLEs included partner losing their job, trouble paying bills, and the death of someone close to the pregnant person. Cannabis use that continued in the postpartum period was significantly associated with the respondents' partner not desiring the pregnancy/child. Additionally, though not categorized as a SLE, intimate partner violence during pregnancy was associated with cannabis use in the perinatal period [7]. Importantly, the overall risk of continuing cannabis use after discovering pregnancy was significantly associated with higher cumulative SLEs endorsed, suggesting a dose-response association between SLEs and cannabis use during pregnancy [7].

Studies examining the impact of adverse childhood experiences (ACEs) show a similar trend. Traditionally research on ACEs has examined the impact of abuse, neglect, or household dysfunction experienced during childhood on adulthood health and health behaviors. Decades of research have firmly established a dose-dependent association of ACEs with a myriad of health conditions including depression, obesity, cardiovascular disease, and cancers [8]. Emerging data have also examined the relationship between ACEs and perinatal mental health. While to date this work has primarily focused on an association between high ACEs and perinatal depression, recent data also suggest that high ACEs are predictive of suicidal thoughts, severe anxiety, and cannabis use during pregnancy. Notably, in one recent study, those who reported six or more ACEs were nearly four times as likely to use cannabis during pregnancy [9].

Clinical Case

Andrea endorses cannabis use daily prior to pregnancy; however, she currently uses 4–5 times per week. She denies alcohol use during pregnancy, excessive caffeine use, and denies use of other substances. She expresses concern that using cannabis will affect her fetus and wants "more than anything to have a healthy baby." She admits that she initially did not want to follow up on her OB's recommendation to see a psychiatrist and is worried about the potential of taking a prescription medication as she has heard those are not safe in pregnancy. However, she does want help for her depression as her mood has been the poorest that she can recall and will not lift with her previous coping skills of calling a friend or going for a walk. Cannabis has been the only thing to help thus far, but even then, she states the effects are temporary and mostly just help with falling asleep. While mood has been her main reason for using cannabis, Andrea states it has also helped with pregnancy-related nausea in the first trimester.

- *What are the most common reasons cited for cannabis use during pregnancy?*
- *How do these factors impact and guide clinical practice?*

Pregnancy-Specific Reasons for Use

Recent data has elucidated reported reasons for using cannabis among pregnant individuals. Chang et al. collected qualitative data on attitudes and beliefs of 25 pregnant women who endorsed cannabis use during pregnancy [10]. Women in this study commonly reported that relief from pregnancy-associated nausea and vomiting, stress management, and/or improved mood were primary motivations for using cannabis. Many of the patients interviewed described beliefs that cannabis was "natural," and therefore perceived as safer to use during pregnancy than other substances (such as tobacco or alcohol) and prescription medications, a finding consistent with previous research. Highlighting the structural component that may contribute to use during pregnancy, one participant noted that cannabis was not only more accessible than mental healthcare, but also more cost-effective. However, overall participants did attempt to reduce use during pregnancy and expressed uncertainty around risks of antenatal cannabis use for their fetus. When the concept of a "natural" substance was challenged with a discussion about tobacco as another natural and plant-derived substance, many interviewees expressed knowledge about the risk tobacco use poses during pregnancy. The lack of data regarding reproductive risk with cannabis use was however interpreted as a lack of risk. This study highlights the importance for continued research on the effects of cannabis use in the perinatal period and clear communication around potential for associated medical and developmental risk [10].

The American College of Obstetrics & Gynecology (ACOG) recommends against cannabis use (as well as other substance use, such as tobacco and alcohol) during pregnancy as well as during the lactation period.

The belief that prescription medications or broader distrust of the medical profession in general is not uncommon and most certainly not unfounded. Medical abuse of disenfranchised or otherwise marginalized and vulnerable populations has long been perpetuated. This underscores the importance of rapport building with patients who have good reason to be apprehensive when seeking medical care and guidance in making health decisions for themselves and their families.

In line with these qualitative data, Young-Wolff et al. recently published a large-scale (n = 196,022 pregnancies) questionnaire-based study in California, a state with legalization of both medicinal and recreational cannabis. They found that cannabis use during pregnancy was associated with higher odds of depression, anxiety, and/or trauma-related diagnoses and symptoms (aOR and 95% CI respectively 2.25 (2.11–2.41), 2.65 (2.46–2.86), and 2.82 (2.59–3.06)) [11]. Further they found that the severity of depression symptoms was positively associated with cannabis use, in a presumably dose-dependent relationship. However, the authors note that further research is ultimately warranted with regard to the impact of cannabis on mood disorders in the setting of pregnancy.

Clinical Case

After a diagnostic evaluation, Andrea is diagnosed with Major Depressive Disorder, recurrent, severe. During the interview she reflects on multiple previous depressive episodes starting in adolescence and often associated with heavier periods of cannabis use. After a comprehensive discussion with the psychiatrist, she would like to consider starting sertraline for depression. While she hopes that this will help her to further reduce cannabis use by improving her mood, she states that she has such a "close relationship with weed" she cannot picture herself maintaining full abstinence. She does very much want to breastfeed her baby and asks for guidance.

- *What evidence exists to guide a discussion with Andrea about lactation?*

Obstetrical and Neonatal Outcomes

THC is highly lipophilic, readily crosses the placenta and into the fetal compartment, and may affect glucose and insulin regulation. Existing data regarding antenatal cannabis use is complicated by confounders (e.g., concurrent tobacco use) and the absence of objective quantitative measures of cannabis exposure. While mixed, data suggest a potential association between antenatal cannabis exposure and small for gestational age infants, preterm birth and stillbirth [12]. Current evidence does not suggest that THC is a human teratogen [12]. Potential neurodevelopmental impacts in the setting of antenatal cannabis use are discussed fully in Chap. 3.

Lactation

Myriad benefits related to breastfeeding for both infant and mother have been well established, and breastfeeding is recognized by the American Academy of Pediatrics (AAP) as the ideal infant feeding method [13]. However, in a setting of a mother who is using cannabis, the benefits of breastfeeding must be considered along with the potential risk of infant exposure. Evidence suggests that chronic cannabis users do not decrease use during lactation and cannabis use is associated with a decreased duration of breastfeeding [14, 15].

THC is highly lipid soluble and has a low molecular weight, properties that allow for easy excretion into breastmilk and accumulation in the infant brain during a period of rapid growth and development [13]. THC is present in breastmilk at concentrations up to eight times that of maternal plasma levels and is absorbed and metabolized by a breastfed infant [15]. As THC is stored in body fat, its elimination from maternal and fetal circulation is variable. Duration of detection in breastmilk ranges from 6 days to over 1 month [16]. At present, no data exists to inform how the concentration of THC in marijuana or the mother's frequency of use is related to the concentration of THC in breastmilk. While THC use is associated with variable changes in levels of prolactin in non-pregnant, non-lactating women, no data exists to suggest that THC use affects breastmilk production [16].

Data regarding infant effects of exposure to cannabinoids via breastmilk is limited and conflicting. While it is well established that exposure to endocannabinoids during times of critical brain development has potential significant and long-lasting effects on cognition and emotion regulation, existing data regarding use in lactation is limited by small sample sizes and confounding factors (e.g., concurrent substance use or sequential exposure to cannabinoids during pregnancy) [17]. Studies conducted decades ago are often cited; however, the potency of THC in available cannabis has increased dramatically since that time and new methods of cannabis use have emerged. While one study suggested that exposure during lactation is associated with delays in infant motor development at 12 months of age, other studies have found no short-term effects on infant growth or development [16]. No data regarding long-term neurodevelopmental effects of exposure to cannabis exclusively during lactation has been reported [17]. Cumulatively, the existing data is considered insufficient to evaluate the effects of exposure to cannabinoids through lactation.

In addition to the potential effects of direct exposure via breastmilk, infants of parents who smoke cannabis are at risk for exposure to secondhand cannabis smoke. THC is present in exhaled breath for up to 2 h after a cannabis cigarette and data suggests that secondhand exposures in adults can be significant [15]. Regardless of method, infant feeding requires frequent and close physical contact with a caretaker. Notably, limited data suggests that infant exposure to secondhand cannabis smoke may be associated with an increased risk of sudden infant death syndrome (SIDS) [17].

Finally, it is important to recognize that when an infant has exposure to cannabis via breastfeeding or secondhand smoke, this exposure likely occurs in the context of parental substance use and potentially along with impaired parenting. Acute effects of cannabis use might include impaired attention, judgment, motor coordination and reaction time. More rarely cannabis use can trigger paranoia or other psychotic symptoms. Long-term regular users may exhibit more persistent changes in executive functioning as well as high-risk behaviors driven by addiction. Parents with substance use disorders more broadly may exhibit dysregulation of the neural stress-reward system and experience interactions with their infant as less rewarding and more stressful [15]. While the impact of maternal cannabis use on infant attachment is poorly understood at this time, broader investigation regarding general substance (i.e., alcohol, cannabis, opiates, etc.) use does support a negative association between perinatal cannabis use and secure dyadic attachment. However, caution advised when interpreting these data as cannabis use (as well as substance use in general) in the perinatal period is also associated with potentially confounding socioeconomic factors that may impact dyadic attachment [18]. Further research on the impact of cannabis use and dyadic attachment is certainly warranted.

Current existing guidelines are clear that cannabis use is not recommended while breastfeeding and that healthcare providers should encourage abstinence from cannabis to breastfeeding individuals [13, 17]. At the present time, however cannabis use is not considered to be an absolute contraindication to breastfeeding and some evidence suggests that lactation care providers are likely to encourage breastfeeding in the setting of cannabis use [19].

Screening

Given the prevalence of cannabis use in the perinatal period, significant barriers to patient self-report, and the potential for harm with fetal or infant exposure, universal screening for cannabis and other substances of abuse is a critical component of perinatal care. As illustrated earlier in this chapter, risk factors for perinatal cannabis use, such as stressful life events, are not easily elucidated within routine obstetrical care and screening based on clinical suspicion risks the incorporation of implicit bias into healthcare practice. All patients should therefore be screened for cannabis along with alcohol, tobacco, and other substances of abuse at the first prenatal visit and at least once per trimester thereafter for those who initially screen positive for current or past use [20]. See Highlights Box 15.1 for commonly used screening tools for substance use in the perinatal period. Of note, while urine drug testing may be a useful adjunctive tool for individuals with substance use disorders, routine urine drug screening (UDS) within obstetrical care has many important limitations. THC can remain positive for long periods of time after cessation in the setting of chronic cannabis use. When used in isolation, UDS cannot provide accurate information about the nature or extent of a patient's use of cannabis or other substances. Furthermore, synthetic cannabinoids (in addition to other drugs of concern such as synthetic opioids) are non-detectable in most standard UDS panels [15, 20]. There is also considerable concern that routine UDS may have negative consequences by negatively impacting the patient–physician relationship and deterring substance-abusing individuals from engaging in prenatal care. Thus it is recommended that UDS not be used as a primary method of screening for substance use in the perinatal period, and only be used with the patient's knowledge and consent [20].

Highlights Box 15.1 Substance Use Screening Tools During the Perinatal Period

- 4Ps
- Substance use profile-Pregnancy
- NIDA Quick Screen *not validated in pregnancy but widely used in practice*

Table 15.1 National Center for Trauma-Informed Care Core Principles and how to incorporate into substance use screening the obstetrical setting

National Center for Trauma-Informed Care Core Principles	Examples of how to implement within obstetrical substance use screening
Trustworthiness and transparency	• Patient is informed about mandatory reporting requirements upfront • Clinician explains that the purpose of screening is to identify need for treatment • Urine drug testing never done without the patient's knowledge
Collaboration and mutuality	• Conversation about substance use focuses on assessment and support of patient's own motivation to change • Treatment planning incorporates patient • Patient is provided with psychoeducation around CUD in pregnancy or lactation in a clear, nonjudgmental and respectful manner
Empowerment, voice and choice	• Urine drug testing done only with patient's consent • When indicated, referral options are provided and treatment plan considers patient's preferences • Discussion around addressing underlying reasons for use

While there are many logistical considerations on *how* to incorporate screening into obstetrical practice, it is critical that clinicians also maintain a purposeful approach to the *patient experience* of the screening process. Certain core principles of trauma-informed care may provide helpful guidance in an effective approach which minimizes risk to the physician–patient relationship and thus the patient's ability to adhere to recommended prenatal and specialty healthcare. These guiding principles along with examples how they may be addressed within the process of perinatal SUD screening process are outlined in Table 15.1.

Finally, while screening itself is likely to increase detection of perinatal substance use, it should be noted that detection itself is not the goal. If a positive screening result is not addressed with an appropriate response, it is of limited value. Screening, brief intervention, and referral to treatment (SBIRT) represents an evidence-based approach to care of substance use disorders within obstetric settings. While SBIRT has been recommended as an approach to perinatal tobacco and alcohol use disorders by the US Preventative Services Task Force and ACOG, evidence supports its use in substance use disorders more broadly as well [20]. Interested readers can see Chap. 4.1 for more information about the SBIRT approach.

Clinical Case

Andrea initiates sertraline and titrates up to 150 mg daily at the advice of her psychiatrist. At 30 weeks gestation she presents to her prenatal care visit and is re-administered the EPDS with a score of 8. Her obstetrician administers as substance use screening tool and notices that Andrea endorses use of cannabis. Upon inquiry, Andrea reports that she has further reduced use to 1–2 "blunts" per week; however, she plans to stop use completely a week prior to her due date as she doesn't want to "test positive" at delivery and risk a report to child protective services.

- *How would Andrea's clinician best approach this concern?*
- *What health or developmental information might be provided to Andrea?*

Legal

Legal requirements around perinatal substance abuse vary significantly by state. Clinicians caring for perinatal patients should therefore be familiar with their states' reporting requirements and potential for criminalization. All US healthcare providers are required to notify child protection officials when caring for an infant affected by substance abuse. Several states also require clinicians to report suspected prenatal substance use and/or test for prenatal exposure if drug use is suspected. Twenty-three states and the District of Columbia consider antenatal substance use as child abuse, and three states consider it as criteria for civil commitment [21]. Importantly, several states have focused on access to treatment by increasing funding for drug treatment programs developed for pregnant persons or prohibiting discrimination based on pregnancy status within publicly funded substance use disorder treatment centers. Readers can reference the Guttmacher Institute for more detailed information on this topic (www.guttmacher.org).

While considerable variability exists among state-based legal approaches to perinatal substance use, guidelines by prominent medical professional organizations are notably similar. The American Academy of Addiction Psychiatry, the American Medical Association, and the American College of Obstetricians and Gynecologists have all issued statements in opposition to criminalization of perinatal substance use and civil commitment. These statements promote a healthcare approach to perinatal substance use which includes patient education, prevention measures, and access to substance use treatment programs [22, 23].

Treatment

Attaining complete abstinence from cannabis can be difficult in the setting of heavy or sustained use and may not be possible for every patient. While concerns around legal implications or social stigma may present as barriers for patients to enter treatment during the perinatal period, pregnancy also presents a unique period of time when patients are likely to have frequent contact with healthcare providers, have insurance coverage and increased overall motivation for optimal health. Of note, evidence suggests pregnant individuals are more aware of the legal repercussions of cannabis use during pregnancy than potential health or developmental risks [10]. Similarly, obstetrical clinicians are more likely to counsel patients on the legal consequences of use rather than health implications [24]. However, cannabis-using pregnant individuals are likely to desire a healthy pregnancy and infant and thus may be further compelled to address problematic substance use by health-focused information [10].

At present no specific pharmacologic treatment is available for cannabis use disorders. While there is no evidence-based approach for treatment specifically within the perinatal period, interventions which have shown effectiveness in the general population are recommended. These include motivation enhancement treatment, contingency management, and cognitive-behavioral therapy [15]. These approaches are discussed in more detail in Chaps. 3.1, 4.1, and 4.2 of this book.

Finally, it is important to note that cannabis use in the perinatal period largely does not happen in isolation. A patient disclosure may serve as a cue to ask more about potential contributing factors such as nausea and vomiting, mood complaints, stressful life circumstances, or interpersonal violence. Individuals who perceive cannabis as a safer alternative to prescription treatments for nausea, depression, or anxiety may be benefit from information about non-pharmacologic treatments for these conditions as well as the overall reassuring reproductive safety profile of commonly used pharmacologic agents. Finally, comprehensive care may require referral to appropriate resources to address critical social determinants of health such as housing assistance, employment services, or domestic violence advocacy.

Clinical Case

With the support of her obstetrical clinician, Andrea successfully enters an outpatient substance use treatment program in the final weeks of her pregnancy and is able to achieve abstinence from cannabis after 4 weeks of treatment. She delivers a baby girl at 39 weeks gestation. As Andrea is in early recovery from cannabis, the obstetrical team does make a referral to child protective services (CPS) at the time of delivery. CPS follows Andrea for the first year of her daughter's life and makes several sequential referrals for resources such as baby supplies, employment services, and parenting supports. While Andrea often experiences CPS monitoring as intrusive and stressful, she reflects that when she does have cravings for cannabis that "someone is going to be looking."

Summary

The prevalence of cannabis use among perinatal individuals has increased significantly in parallel with the general population. The commercialization of cannabis has both complicated its study and contributed to a public perception of cannabis as a "natural" alternative to traditional treatments for physical symptoms or medical conditions, inclusive of pregnancy-related concerns. While emerging data suggest that cannabis is a substance of concern in the perinatal period, further research in this area is a critical need. Perinatal healthcare clinicians have a unique opportunity to implement recommended screening for substance use as a routine component of perinatal care in a manner that prioritizes the physician–patient relationship and the provision of evidence-based information and treatments.

Highlights Box 15.2 Key Points in Treatment and Management

- The prevalence of cannabis us has increased in recent years in the general population as well as in perinatal individuals.
- Commonly stated reasons for cannabis use in pregnancy include nausea and vomiting, mood complaints, and coping with stress.
- Universal screening for cannabis use during the perinatal period should be implemented in a way that maintains transparency and prioritizes the patient–physician relationship.
- Patients should be provided with clear guidance of health information regarding cannabis use during pregnancy and postpartum as well as information about healthcare provider reporting requirements.
- Patients should be counseled to not use cannabis during pregnancy or lactation.
- Treatment planning in the context of perinatal cannabis use should be comprehensive and patient-centered.

References

1. United Nations. United Nations: World Drug Report 2019; 2020.
2. SAMHSA. 2019 National Survey on drug use and health: women [internet]. US Department of Health and Human Services; 2020 [cited 2021 Jun 30]. https://www.samhsa.gov/data/sites/default/files/reports/rpt31102/2019NSDUH-Women/Women%202019%20NSDUH.pdf.
3. Volkow ND, Han B, Compton WM, McCance-Katz EF. Self-reported medical and nonmedical cannabis use among pregnant women in the United States. JAMA. 2019;322(2):167–9.
4. Murray RM, Hall W. Will legalization and commercialization of cannabis use increase the incidence and prevalence of psychosis?. JAMA psychiatry. 2020;77(8):777–8.
5. Brown QL, Sarvet AL, Shmulewitz D, Martins SS, Wall MM, Hasin DS. Trends in marijuana use among pregnant and nonpregnant reproductive-aged women, 2002–2014. Jama. 2017;317(2):207–9.
6. Ko JY, Coy KC, Haight SC, Haegerich TM, Williams L, Cox S, Njai R, Grant AM. Characteristics of marijuana use during pregnancy—eight states, pregnancy risk assessment monitoring system, 2017. Morbidity and mortality weekly report. 2020;69(32):1058.

7. Allen AM, Jung AM, Alexander AC, Allen SS, Ward KD, al'Absi M. Cannabis use and stressful life events during the perinatal period: cross-sectional results from pregnancy risk assessment monitoring system (PRAMS) data, 2016. Addiction. 2020;115(9):1707–16.
8. Merrick MT, Ford DC, Ports KA, Guinn AS, Chen J, Klevens J, Metzler M, Jones CM, Simon TR, Daniel VM, Ottley P. Vital signs: Estimated proportion of adult health problems attributable to adverse childhood experiences and implications for prevention—25 States, 2015–2017. Morbidity and Mortality Weekly Report. 2019;68(44):999.
9. Jasthi DL, Nagle-Yang S, Frank S, Masotya M, Huth-Bocks A. Associations between adverse childhood experiences and prenatal mental health and substance use among urban, low-income women. Community Ment Health J [Internet]; 2021 Jun 28 [cited 2021 Jun 30]. https://link.springer.com/10.1007/s10597-021-00862-1.
10. Chang JC, Tarr JA, Holland CL, De Genna NM, Richardson GA, Rodriguez KL, et al. Beliefs and attitudes regarding prenatal marijuana use: perspectives of pregnant women who report use. Drug Alcohol Depend. 2019;1(196):14–20.
11. Young-Wolff KC, Silver LD, Brown QL. Moving toward health and social equity for women who use cannabis during preconception, pregnancy, and lactation. JAMA Netw Open. 2021;4(2):e210148.
12. Metz TD, Stickrath EH. Marijuana use in pregnancy and lactation: a review of the evidence. Am J Obstet Gynecol. 2015;213(6):761–78.
13. Ryan SA, Ammerman SD, O'Connor ME, Committee on Substance Use and Prevention; Section on Breastfeeding SO. Marijuana use during pregnancy and Breastfeeding: implications for neonatal and childhood outcomes. Pediatrics [Internet]; 2018 Sep 1 [cited 2021 Mar 14];142(3). https://pediatrics.aappublications.org/content/142/3/e20181889.
14. Crume TL, Juhl AL, Brooks-Russell A, Hall KE, Wymore E, Borgelt LM. Cannabis use during the perinatal period in a state with legalized recreational and medical marijuana: the association between maternal characteristics, Breastfeeding patterns, and neonatal outcomes. J Pediatr. 2018;197:90–6.
15. Velez ML, Jordan CJ, Jansson LM. Cannabis use disorder during the perinatal period. In: Montoya ID, Weiss SRB, editors. Cannabis use disorders [Internet]. Cham: Springer; 2019 [cited 2021 March 14]. p. 177–88. https://doi.org/10.1007/978-3-319-90365-1_17.
16. Drugs and Lactation Database (LactMed) [Internet]. Cannabis. [Internet]. National Library of Medicine (US); 2006 [cited 2021 Apr 1]. https://www.ncbi.nlm.nih.gov/books/NBK501587/.
17. Reece-Stremtan S, Marinelli KA. ABM clinical protocol #21: guidelines for breastfeeding and substance use or substance use disorder, revised 2015. Breastfeed Med. 2015;10(3):135–41.
18. Hyysalo N, Gastelle M, Flykt M. Maternal pre-and postnatal substance use and attachment in young children: A systematic review and meta-analysis. Development and Psychopathology. 2021;16:1–8.
19. Brandt L, Leifheit AK, Finnegan LP, Fischer G. Management of substance abuse in pregnancy: maternal and neonatal aspects. In: Psychopharmacology and pregnancy. Cham: Springer; 2014. p. 169–95.
20. Wright TE, Terplan M, Ondersma SJ, Boyce C, Yonkers K, Chang G, et al. The role of screening, brief intervention, and referral to treatment in the perinatal period. Am J Obstet Gynecol. 2016;215(5):539–47.
21. Guttmacher Institute. Substance use during pregnancy: state laws and policies [Internet]; 2021 [cited 2021 Jun 30]. https://www.guttmacher.org/state-policy/explore/substance-use-during-pregnancy.
22. American College of Obstetricians Gynecologists. Committee opinion No. 473: substance abuse reporting and pregnancy: the role of the obstetrician–gynecologist. Obstet Gynecol. 2011;117(1):200–1.
23. House SJ, Coker JL, Stowe ZN. Perinatal substance abuse: at the clinical crossroads of policy and practice. Am J Psychiatry. 2016;173(11):1077–80.
24. Holland CL, Rubio D, Rodriguez KL, Kraemer KL, Day N, Arnold RM, et al. Obstetric health care providers' counseling responses to pregnant patient disclosures of marijuana use. Obstet Gynecol. 2016;127(4):681–7.

Cannabis in the Geriatric Population 16

Helena Winston

Geriatric Populations and Cannabis

Case

Mr. Gerison is an 80-year-old former lawyer with a past medical history of chronic low back pain, chronic obstructive pulmonary disease (COPD), coronary artery disease, hypertension, and insomnia who is admitted to the hospital with confusion after a fall. He also has a history of glaucoma that has been treated by his ophthalmologist with cannabis in the past. He takes multiple medications as prescribed, including doxepin 10 mg for sleep, lisinopril 40 mg, amlodipine 10 mg, and various inhaled medications for his COPD, all of which he has been taking for 15 years. He is currently afebrile with vital signs, CMP, CBC, and CT head all within normal limits. He has no history of illicit drug use of any kind, except once trying a joint back in the sixties, and has never smoked cigarettes. He rarely drinks alcohol. He appears confused and according to his wife, has not been sleeping well for years despite seeing a sleep specialist and trying all recommended medications and behavioral therapies, including sleep hygiene and cognitive behavioral therapy for insomnia (CBT-I). Consultation-liaison psychiatry is consulted and determines that about a year ago, one of Mr. Gerison's friends recommended he see a provider regarding medical marijuana and he started taking THC/CBD gummies to help him fall asleep. He felt that it was useful. About a month ago he decided to try a different type of marijuana for his chronic low back pain. He thought about smoking flower but wanted to avoid carcinogens so instead decided to start vaping.

H. Winston (✉)
Department of Psychiatry, University of Colorado, School of Medicine, Aurora, CO, USA

Denver Health, Denver, CO, USA
e-mail: Helena.Winston@CUAnschutz.edu

P. Riggs, T. Thant (eds.), *Cannabis in Psychiatric Practice*, Psychiatry Update 3,
https://doi.org/10.1007/978-3-031-04874-6_16

Introduction and Literature Review

The "elderly" are a diverse population generally defined as those 65 years of age or older. Falls and confusion are common in this group and risk increases with age, frailty, comorbidities, and polypharmacy. But how does cannabis use complicate the picture? Mr. Gerison takes THC/CBD gummies for sleep and started vaping marijuana for chronic low back pain—given his age, how might cannabis possibly affect him? There is fairly little research on cannabis and the elderly, although there has been an increase in the number of papers published on cannabis use in this age group over time, with a change in cumulative total numbers of papers published of about +180 in 2017 compared to around 2000 [1].

Trends in Use

From 2015 to 2018 there was a 75% relative increase in the prevalence of marijuana use by adults 65 years and older [2, 3]. From 2002 to 2014, use among those 65 and old increased 333% (the second greatest percent increase of any age group—the first being those aged 55–64) [4]. Cannabis is also the most frequently used non-prescribed or "illicit" drug consumed among the elderly [5], so it should not be a surprise that Mr. Gerison is using cannabis products. A 2018 study reported that 2.9% of those 65 years and older used marijuana in the past year [6]. This exceeded the projections of a 2006 study that hypothesized that the number of people 50 and older using marijuana in the past year would increase to 2.9% by 2020, years later than what has actually occurred [7]. An anonymous survey of 568 elderly individuals in a geriatrics clinic found that 15% had used marijuana in the past 3 years, 53% used regularly (weekly or daily), 61% used it for the first time when they were 61 years or older, and 46% used cannabidiol-only substances [8]. A survey of 345 patients in two academic geriatrics clinics in Colorado found that 32% had used cannabis in the past, more than 50% were 75 years or older, about 25% were 85 years and older, and most were white women. Only 9 people reported negative side effects [9]. The elderly's perceptions of marijuana also differ somewhat from younger groups, and they may perceive the effects of marijuana more negatively than those aged 18–34, but evidence is mixed. For example, 32% of the elderly think marijuana is very addictive, while only 22% of the younger age group believes the same thing. Similarly, 41% of the elderly think smoking 1 joint a day is much less safe than drinking 1 glass of wine per day, as compared to 25% of the younger group thinking the same thing [10]. A contrasting study however found that people over 50 were more likely than middle-aged (30–49 years old) or young people (18–29 years old) to think that marijuana was not addictive and that marijuana cessation would not be problematic [11]. Mr. Gerison tried marijuana when he was fairly young, as per some studies, geriatric marijuana users first used it before age 18 [5]. That said, a recent study of over 550 geriatric adults noted that 61% used marijuana for the first time during or after age 61. Mr. Gerison tried it once in the sixties and may now be seeing his friends try it in their old age. He may have conflicting opinions about marijuana use and view it as a medicinal, not recreational substance.

Metabolism of THC in the Elderly

The geriatric population in general has decreased hepatic metabolism, renal blood flow and clearance, and muscle mass, and increased gastrointestinal transit time, all of which affect drug absorption, processing, and elimination and can contribute to plasma levels, drug–drug interactions, and adverse side effects. Decreased fat content, which can be occur in some of the elderly, may increase the clinical immediate effect of cannabis in this population. However, over one-third of those over 65 were considered obese as of a 2012 study [12]. Those with increased fat may have a detectable blood level—and thus effects—for longer, even after cessation, as THC is lipophilic and dissolves in lipoid tissue. As a result, many clinicians choose to give the elderly low doses of medications and try to reduce polypharmacy as much as possible. As mentioned in other chapters, cannabis may cause CYP450 inhibition in the liver further raising the blood levels of other medications. In Mr. Gerison's case, cannabis may have raised the levels of one of his other medications, increasing his risk of falling and confusion.

There is little data regarding drug–drug interactions with marijuana or the processing of THC itself in the elderly population. THC trials have generally not included research on this group of people, although there is one small phase 1 randomized double-blind placebo-controlled crossover trial that compared the effect of three dosages (3 mg, 5 mg, 6.5 mg) of oral tablet THC in 11 cannabis-naïve elderly adults (age range 65–80 years old) [13]. It found that overall THC was safe and well tolerated even when combined with other medications. Adverse events, when they occurred (most frequently somnolence 27% or dry mouth 11%), increased with dosage amount [13]. Coordination problems (7%), impaired concentration (7%), blurry vision (5%), dizziness (5%), and visual hallucinations (2%), among other side effects, also occurred, and such side effects may increase the risk of falls or confusion, as seen with Mr. Gerison. The study also found that THC pharmacokinetics such as plasma concentration varied widely between individual subjects, suggesting that in the elderly THC may have variable effects depending on the individual. Pharmacodynamics (actual effects) of THC were however surprisingly low as the study subjects rarely felt "high" with these doses and "body sway" was no different than with placebo [13].

Falls, Cannabis, and the Elderly

The risk of falling and the seriousness of fall sequelae increase with age due to increased frailty, decreasing bone mass, and impaired wound healing. In 2015, over $50 billion was spent in the USA on fatal and non-fatal falls in the elderly [14]. Mr. Gerison had a fall. This may have been due to risk factors like older age, polypharmacy, or being on anti-hypertensive medications. That said, cannabis may also have played a role. There is some evidence that in older adults (50 years and older), marijuana use is associated with injury and injury is associated with ED visits [15]. Cannabinoid receptors (CB1) are distributed throughout the cerebellum and as such there is evidence to suspect that in addition to marijuana acutely impairing memory, attention, and executive function, it also impairs coordinated activities such as walking or negotiating stairs [16]. In a study of 350 homeless adults 50 years and older (who often have the added fall risks of being in unsafe environments and overall poor health), one-third reported a fall in the past 6 months at baseline. In follow-up assessments, it was determined that about 39% used marijuana and that marijuana use (among other things) was associated with an increased risk of falls in this population [17]. Meanwhile, a 2021 study matched a total of 16 marijuana users and non-users and found that users had slower gaits and were less able to balance on one leg suggesting that marijuana impaired these faculties leading to a documented increased risk of falling [18]. Mr. Gerison's use of vaping products in addition to this THC/CBD gummies for sleep, may have impaired his balance and coordination leading to his fall.

Driving, Cannabis, and the Elderly

Older people may not be aware that cannabis might worsen their ability to drive a vehicle. It may be worth talking to Mr. Gerison about if and how much he drives and the potential effects of cannabis use on driving. Cannabis likely impairs the faculties, such as short-term memory, attention, executive function, and motor coordination required for driving, and increases the risk of motor vehicle collisions [16]. Reaction time decreases and lane weaving increases with cannabis use, raising the risk of motor vehicle accident involvement by 2× [19]. Many elderly people are afraid of losing their driver's license; if they are educated as to the effects that cannabis may have on their driving skills and risk of accidents, this may alter their use patterns.

Dementia and Cannabis

Cannabis can cause cognitive slowing, which may be difficult to disentangle from cognitive decline, especially in those with chronic or heavy cannabis use. Similarly, the symptoms of major neurocognitive disorder (e.g., Alzheimer's disease) in the elderly can be confused with *acute confusion* or *mood problems*. Time course is essential in helping to narrow down the diagnosis. An evaluation of oral intake, sleep changes and medications, basic lab workup, and potential imaging, as well as a good history from family and friends can help rule out acute causes of confusion and altered mental status. In Mr. Gerison's case, his confusion appears to have been fairly acute in onset and after reviewing the chart, basic causes of confusion such as hypoxia, infection, electrolyte abnormalities, bleeds, and stroke have been ruled out. However, could Mr. Gerison be showing signs of pseudodementia? The amount of effort he puts forth in basic or extensive cognitive screening tests may help clarify the picture, with more effort usually signally dementia as opposed to depression (which is often accompanied by apathy). But what about the marijuana? In one study of adults 60 and older seeking outpatient psychiatric care, of those who met criteria for depression, cannabis was used by 12% of men and 4% of women in the past month. Thus many people who are depressed may be using marijuana and cognitive decrements due to marijuana may confound the depression picture [20]. As a consultation-liaison psychiatrist it is thus important to be aware of the potential acute and long-term cognitive effects of cannabis.

It is unknown whether cannabis use when young contributes to the development of neurocognitive disorders in older age. Mr. Gerison just started using cannabis in the last year, and duration of use has not been substantial. It is unlikely that cannabis has caused sudden onset of major neurocognitive disorder; however, Mr. Gerison does have risk factors for dementia and no studies exist tracing onset of use as an older adult and the effects of cannabis on dementia. Cannabis is known to acutely impair short-term memory, procedural memory, working memory, memory acquisition, and sensory perception, among other aspects of cognition [21], which may or may not exacerbate age-related declines in memory and cognition [21] as long-term study data is lacking [22].

Marijuana is also being used to *treat* dementia. There are ten states in which dementia (especially agitation in Alzheimer's disease [AD]) is considered a qualifying condition for medical marijuana; however, evidence for use at best remains unclear [23]. In 2010, a review of then existent literature found 80 articles on dementia and marijuana. Many of these studies suggested a role for the endocannabinoid system in the neurobiology of dementia, however, there was little in vivo confirmation of in vitro studies [24]. A 2019 systematic analysis found nine studies involving CBD or THC and AD that could be analyzed quantitatively. These in vitro and in vivo studies indicated a potential role for these compounds in treating AD [25]. Then, in 2020, Fernández-Ruiz et al. [26] outlined the research on THC for dementia and summarized that while animal studies are somewhat promising (e.g., stimulation of the CB1 receptor can decrease the formation of amyloid plaques and neurofibrillary tangles—common findings in Alzheimer's disease), human studies are less so. This article pointed out that clinical studies vary in design and outcomes, and also have a fairly substantial risk of bias. Recent evidence for the use of cannabinoids in dementia remains mixed. The authors reviewed recent studies and found that some randomized double-blind placebo-controlled crossover studies suggest that delta9-THC does not affect the neuropsychiatric symptoms of Alzheimer's disease, including agitation, aggression, anxiety, or falls, among others, or affect activities of daily living (ADLs) and quality of life (QOL) (research by Van Den Elsen et al. from 2015 and 2017) [27, 28, 29]. By contrast, a 2019 randomized, double-blind crossover study versus placebo suggests that nabilone improves agitation in those with Alzheimer's disease (research by Hermann et al. 2019) [30]. Meanwhile, a study of *self-reported* cognition in older adults (≥50) exposed to marijuana, found variable effects that suggested that longer duration and quantity of use was associated with poorer cognition but not universally so, indicating that objective studies are needed [31].

Insomnia, Cannabis, and the Elderly

Insomnia is one of the main reasons that elderly people turn to cannabis. In survey of 345 people treated at geriatric primary care clinics, 38% used marijuana for sleep and sleep was the second most common reason for marijuana use in this age group [9]. In a much smaller Canadian convenience sample qualitative study that focused on adults aged 71–85, half of the 12 participants used marijuana for sleep [32]. Evidence for the actual benefit of cannabis on sleep is unclear. A small study exploring the effects of cannabis on sleep in older adults with and without HIV found that cannabis use increased total sleep time in both populations [33].

Another found that dronabinol may be helpful for nighttime agitation interfering with sleep in those with severe dementia [34]. Overall however more substantive data is lacking.

Chronic Pain, Cannabis, and the Elderly

Mr. Gerison started vaping marijuana to help treat his pain. Between 2000 and 2017, there were 179 papers published on cannabis and chronic pain [1] and pain is one of the prime indications for which individuals report using marijuana derivatives. A prospective study examined 2736 patients over 65 years old receiving cannabis (mostly for chronic pain or cancer) in a specialized medical cannabis clinic and found that after 6 months of treatment, almost 94% felt their pain was greatly reduced and 18.1% had reduced the dose of or stopped opioids [35]. Overall, prescribed marijuana may reduce pain by 30%, including in older adults needing palliative care [36]. That said, the concentrates used in vape pens can vary considerably in amount of THC and Mr. Gerison may have been using far more than he had intended leading to acute mental status changes and impaired coordination as outlined above.

Other Cannabis Usage in the Elderly

The elderly report using cannabis derivatives for many reasons (Tables 16.1 and 16.2) and studies on efficacy remain uncertain (Table 16.2). Of 105 papers investigating the effects of cannabinoids in the elderly, none showed efficacy in treating shortness of breath, dyskinesia, nausea, and emesis due to chemotherapy and only two studies suggested possible use in anorexia and neuropsychiatric symptoms of dementia [37]. There are guidelines published by The Canadian Agency for Drugs and Technologies in Health (CADTH) that review the medical uses of cannabis in palliative care [38] and largely find the evidence to be mixed and insufficient at this time.

Table 16.1 Reasons for marijuana use in the elderly

Anxiety
Appetite stimulation
Dementia
Depression
Emesis or gastrointestinal distress
Glaucoma
Insomnia or other sleep disturbance
Libido
Memory aid
Migraine
Pain, arthritis especially
Post-traumatic stress disorder
Recreational use
Seizure

Summarized from Yang et al. [8] and Reynolds et al. [9], with modifications
Bolded text: most common

Table 16.2 Results of a study of geriatric individuals perceiving positive marijuana benefit on indicated symptoms ($n = 345$)

	% using cannabis for named indication	% of those perceiving benefit
1. Anxiety	24	100
2. Depression	22	92
3. Sleep	38	86
4. Pain	64	83
5. PTSD	11	50
6. Memory	16	44
7. Migraines	13	14

Adapted from [9], Table 2 and Figure 1

Overall it appears that the evidence for the use of cannabis derivatives in dementia is still unclear and providers should remain cautious, despite individual positive and negative studies. For example, in 2020, another review of the literature reported that mixed quality evidence indicates that there is no clear use for cannabis in reducing the symptoms of dementia and that a total of only 117 people have been studied in randomized controlled trials [36].

Treatment Approaches

Mr. Gerison is on multiple medications, some of which were named in the case. Polypharmacy greatly increases the risk of drug–drug interactions, adverse events, and side effects such as confusion and falls. The effects of cannabis derivatives on medications is largely unknown although cannabis can impact the CYP450 enzymes and, because it itself is processed by the same enzyme set, can be affected by other medications. Thus cannabis levels can be raised or lowered by other medications and cannabis can raise or lower other medication levels. Counseling a patient on the unknown effects of cannabis and other medications is important in helping the patient to make informed decisions.

When interviewing an elderly patient it is also important to gather a thorough history of all medications and over the counter substances being used, including marijuana and gummies. Use lots of terms such as CBD or THC candies, gummies, edibles, wax, shatter, flower, bud, etc. There are innumerable terms for marijuana products and the elderly may not think you are asking about their CBD lozenge when you ask about marijuana usage. Also ask about mechanism of use; some people like Mr. Gerison may think that vaping is safer than smoking marijuana and may not be aware of the increased concentrations often administered through vape pens, as well as the increased risk of psychotic side effects. Many people in states in which cannabis is legal may not even consider cannabis a "drug" and not even think about it when asked if they use any substances. Be specific. Do you use any marijuana, cannabis, or CBD products? How? How much? What for?

Remember to be cognizant of preconceptions about the elderly when interviewing older individuals. You might assume that a laid-back hippie who attended free love festivals in the 1960s is smoking marijuana (and you may or may not be correct!) but you might not think that a strait-laced former lawyer who rarely even drinks alcohol is using cannabis products. Try to free yourself from the stigma that have been associated with drug use. Marijuana is becoming more like alcohol and in some hospitals in states where it is legal, urine drug screens do not even test for it (they assume everyone is using it). Mr. Gerison had received glaucoma treatment with cannabis products and his family friend recommended an evaluation for what is termed "medical" marijuana. Mr. Gerison likely sees his CBD/THC gummies like melatonin gummies and his vaping a bit like COPD inhaled treatments. Be sure however to look for signs and symptoms of use disorders including negative effects on relationships, increasing use, withdrawal, and tolerance levels. It is never wrong to screen for a substance use disorder as these can be of insidious onset, especially when begun via licit channels.

Mr. Gerison has used marijuana products for insomnia for about 1 year and has been vaping marijuana for chronic back pain for a couple of months. He seems to have done fairly well without falls or cognition problems until he started vaping. Having a discussion with him about the amount, concentration, and mode of marijuana use will likely be useful in helping him and his wife make informed decisions moving forward.

Conclusion

Mr. Gerison's case highlights multiple aspects of cannabis use in the elderly. Physiologic changes in the elderly may affect the pharmacokinetics and dynamics of cannabis, and alter drug–drug interactions. Because the elderly are often on multiple medications, cannabis may exacerbate the risks of polypharmacy. The geriatric population may not perceive cannabis as a "drug," especially if they are receiving "medical marijuana." They similarly may not recognize the signs of abuse or dependence. The elderly use cannabis products for a variety of reasons, the evidence for which is stronger with regard to some (like chronic pain or cancer) than others (anxiety or symptoms of dementia); although perceived benefit may be much different. Making sure your patients are appraised of the state of the literature and research is important in helping them to make good and informed choices, especially in states where marijuana use is legal.

Highlights Box 16.1 Key Points for Patient Psychoeducation

- The number of elderly people (65 years and older) using marijuana products is steadily increasing.
- Elderly people process medications and substances such as cannabis differently than younger individuals, and the pharmacokinetics and pharmacodynamics have not been well studied in this population.

- Marijuana impairs short-term memory, executive functioning, decision-making, abstract reasoning, and coordination/reaction time and thus could increase fall risk or driving accidents.
- Per the American Psychiatric Association policy statement there is currently no indication for cannabis as a treatment for any psychiatric disorder [39].
- There is some evidence that marijuana products increase the risk of falls, and thus fractures, in the elderly. Marijuana may also increase the elderly's risk of motor vehicle collisions.
- Geriatric individuals often use marijuana products to treat insomnia or other sleep disturbances and chronic pain. There is some evidence that it is perceived as useful for these conditions.

Highlights Box 16.2 Key Points in Treatment and Management

- Try to keep assumptions at bay. The elderly may be using more or less cannabis than you assume.
- Focus on education and informed decision-making. Older persons may not know the full risks and benefits of marijuana-derived products or they may assume the risks are the same as they were back in the 1960s.
- Realize that there is some evidence for the use of marijuana to treat chronic pain and insomnia, two of the major reasons that the elderly often use to use cannabis. Point out that the evidence for the use of cannabis in dementia is very limited.
- Use caution when recommending cannabis-derived products to the elderly, even for approved indications, and make sure to stress that drug–drug interactions are largely unknown.

References

1. Treister-Goltzman Y, Freud T, Press Y, Peleg R. Trends in publications on medical cannabis from the year 2000. Popul Health Manag. 2019;22(4):362–8.
2. Han BH, Palamar JJ. Trends in cannabis use among older adults in the United States, 2015-2018. JAMA Intern Med. 2020;180(4):609–11.
3. Ahamed A, Kullmann KC, Frasso R, Goldstein JN. Trends in cannabis use among older adults in the United States, 2015–2018. JAMA Intern Med. 2020;180(4):609–11.
4. Azofeifa A, Mattson ME, Schauer G, McAfee T, Grant A, Lyerla R. National estimates of marijuana use and related indicators: National Survey on Drug Use and Health, United States, 2002–2014. CDC MMWR Surveill Summ. 2016;65(11):1–25.
5. Lloyd SL, Striley CW. Marijuana use among adults 50 years or older in the 21st century. Gerontol Geriatr Med. 2018;4:2333721418781668.
6. Han BH, Palamar JJ. Marijuana use by middle aged and older adults in the United States, 2015-2016. Drug Alcohol Depend. 2018;191:374–81.

7. Colliver JD, Compton WM, Gfroerer JC, Condon T. Projecting drug use among aging baby boomers in 2020. Ann Epidemiol. 2006;16:257–65.
8. Yang KH, Kaufmann CN, Nafsu R, Lifset ET, Nguyen K, Sexton M, Han BH, Kim A, Moore AA. Cannabis: an emerging treatment for common symptoms in older adults. J Am Geriatr Sci. 2021;69:91–7.
9. Reynolds IR, Fixen DR, Parnes BL, Lum HD, Shanbhag P, Church S, Linnebur SA, Orosz G. Characteristics and patterns of marijuana use in community-dwelling older adults. J Am Geriatr Sci. 2018;66:2167–71.
10. Keyhani S, Steigerwald S, Ishida J, Vali M, Cerdá M, Hasin D, Dollinger C, Yoo SR, Cohen BE. Risks and benefits of marijuana use: a national survey of U.S. adults. Ann Intern Med. 2018;169(5):282–92.
11. Sexton M, Cuttler C, Mischley LK. A survey of cannabis acute effects and withdrawal symptoms: differential responses across user types and age. J Altern Complement Med. 2019;25(3):326–35.
12. Fakhouri THI, Ogden CL, Carroll MD, Kit BK, Flegal KM. Prevalence of obesity among older adults in the United States, 2007–2010. NCHS Data Brief No. 106; September 2012. https://www.cdc.gov/nchs/products/databriefs/db106.htm.
13. Ahmed AIA, van den Elsen GAH, Colbers A, van der Marck MA, Burger DM, Feuth TB, Olde Rikkert MGM, Kramers C. Safety and pharmacokinetics of oral delta-9-tetrahydrocannabinol in healthy older subjects: a randomized controlled trial. Eur Neuropsychopharmacol. 2014;24:1475–82.
14. Florence CS, Bergen G, Atherly A, Burns E, Stevens J, Drake C. Medical costs of fatal and nonfatal falls in older adults. J Am Geriatr Sci. 2018;66:693–8.
15. Choi NG, Nathan Marti C, DiNitto DM, Choi BY. Older adults' marijuana use, injuries, and emergency department visits. The American Journal of Drug and Alcohol Abuse. 2018;44(2):215–23.
16. Solomon HV, Greenstein AP, DeLisi LE. Cannabis use in older adults: a perspective. Harv Rev Psychiatry. 2021;29:225.
17. Abbs E, Brown R, Guzman D, Kaplan L, Kushel M. Risk factors for falls in older adults experiencing homelessness: results from the HOPE HOME Cohort Study. J Gen Intern Med. 2020;35(6):1813–20.
18. Workman CD, Fietsam AC, Sosnoff J, Rudroff T. Increased likelihood of falling in older cannabis users vs. non-users. Brain Sci. 2021;(11)134.
19. Hartman RL, Huestis MA. Cannabis effects on driving skills. Clin Chem. 2013;59(3):478. https://doi.org/10.1373/clinchem.2012.194381.
20. Satre DD, Sterling SA, Mackin RS, Weisner C. Patterns of alcohol and drug use among depressed older adults seeking outpatient psychiatric services. Am J Geriatr Psychiatry. 2011;19(8):695–703.
21. Sachs J, McGlade E, Yurgelun-Todd D. Safety and toxicology of cannabinoids. Neurotherapeutics. 2015;12:735–46.
22. Weinstein G, Sznitman SR. The implications of late-late cannabis use on brain health: a mapping review and implications for future research. Ageing Res Rev. 2020;59:101041.
23. Maust DT, Bonar EE, Ilgen MA, Blow FC, Kales HC. Agitation in Alzheimer disease as a qualifying condition for medical marijuana in the United States. J Geriatr Psychiatry. 2016;24:1000–3.
24. Walther S, Halpern M. Cannabinoids and dementia: a review of clinical and preclinical data. Pharmaceuticals. 2010;3:2689–708.
25. Kim SH, Yang JW, Kim KH, Kim JU, Yook TH. A review on studies of marijuana for Alzheimer's disease: focusing on CBD, THC. J Pharmacopunct. 2019;22(4):225–30.
26. Fernández-Ruiz J, Galve-Roperh I, Sagredo O, Guzmán M. Possible therapeutic applications of cannabis in the neuropsychopharmacology field. Eur Neuropsychopharmacol. 2020;36:217–34.

27. Van Den Elsen GAH, Ahmed AIA, Verkes RJ, Feuth T, Van Der Marck MA, Olde Rikkert MGM. Tetrahydro-cannabinol in behavioral disturbances in dementia: a crossover randomized controlled trial. Am J Geriatr Psychiatry. 2015a;23:1214–24.
28. Van Den Elsen GAH, Ahmed AIA, Verkes RJ, Kramers C, Feuth T, Rosenberg PB, Van Der Marck MA, Olde Rikkert MGM. Tetrahydrocannabinol for neuropsychiatric symptoms in dementia: a randomized controlled trial. Neurology. 2015b;84:2338–46.
29. Van Den Elsen GAH, Tobben L, Ahmed AIA, Verkes RJ, Kramers C, Marijnissen RM, Olde Rikkert MGM, Van Der Marck MA. Effects of tetrahydrocannabinol on balance and gait in patients with dementia: a randomised controlled crossover trial. J Psychopharmacol. 2017;31(2):184–91. https://doi.org/10.1177/0269881116665357. Epub 2016 Sep 27.
30. Hermann N, Ruthirakuhan M, Gallagher D, Verhoeff NPLG, Kiss A, Black SE, Lanctot KL. Randomized placebo-controlled trial of nabilone for agitation in Alzheimer's disease. Am J Geriatr Psychiatry. 2019;(11):1161–73.
31. Benitez A, Lauzon S, Nietert PJ, McRae-Clark A, Sherman BJ. Self-reported cognition and marijuana use in older adults: results from the national epidemiologic survey on alcohol and related conditions-III. Addict Behav. 2020;108:106437.
32. Baumbusch J, Yip IS. Exploring new use of cannabis among older adults. Clin Gerontol. 2021;44(1):25–31.
33. Campbell LM, Tang B, Watson CW-M, Higgins M, Cherner M, Henry BL, Moore RC. Cannabis use is associated with greater total sleep time in middle-aged and older adults with and without HIV: a preliminary report utilizing digital health technologies. Can Underwrit. 2020;3(2):180–9. https://doi.org/10.26828/cannabis.2020.02.005.
34. Walther S, Mahlberg R, Eichmann U, Kunz D. Delta-9-tetrahydrocannabinol for nighttime agitation in severe dementia. Psychopharmacology. 2006;185:524–8.
35. Abuhasira R, Schleider LB-L, Mechoulam R, Novack V. Epidemiological characteristics, safety and efficacy of medical cannabis in the elderly. Eur J Intern Med. 2018;49:44–50.
36. Levy C, Galenbeck E, Magid K. Cannabis for symptom management in older adults. Med Clin N Am. 2020;104:471–89.
37. van den Elsen GAH, Ahmed AIA, Lammers M, Kramers C, Verkes RJ, van der Marck MA, Olde Rikkert MGM. Efficacy and safety of medical cannabinoids in older subjects: a systematic review. Ageing Res Rev. 2014;14:56–64.
38. MacDonald E, Farrah K. Medical cannabis use in palliative care: review of clinical effectiveness and guidelines: an update. Ottawa: CADTH; 2019. (CADTH rapid response report: summary with critical appraisal).
39. American Psychiatric Association. Position statement in opposition to cannabis as medicine. 2019. https://www.psychiatry.org/File%20Library/About-APA/Organization-Documents-Policies/Policies/Position-Cannabis-as-Medicine.pdf.

Marijuana Use in Organ Transplantation 17

Gerald Scott Winder and Erin G. Clifton

Clinical Case

"Dave" is a 37-year-old male with end-stage renal disease secondary to type I diabetes who is being evaluated for kidney transplant. Transplant social work has concerns about his mood, anxiety, and substance use which prompted a referral to transplant psychiatry. At evaluation outset, Dave states that he's unhappy about seeing a psychiatrist and is unclear why it is necessary. His guardedness lessens with rapport.

Dave has had "attacks" of anger and anxiety for years. Several sessions of counseling were unhelpful 15 years ago and he has since found that daily smoked marijuana and 2 mg of alprazolam, a dose he frequently exceeds, have been more helpful with his emotions. He smokes a half pack of cigarettes per day. Dave has a remote history of using other recreational substances, including cocaine and methamphetamine, which resulted in several substance-related legal consequences. Dave disagrees with psychiatry's recommendations to judiciously taper alprazolam and marijuana and pursue other pharmacological and psychotherapeutic treatment options for mood and anxiety. After being asked to stop at the lab before leaving the clinic, Dave leaves the clinic without providing a urine sample for toxicology.

While the kidney selection committee does not have a firm policy against marijuana, they close Dave's transplant evaluation due to concerns about

G. S. Winder (✉)
Department of Psychiatry, University of Michigan, Ann Arbor, MI, USA

Department of Surgery, University of Michigan, Ann Arbor, MI, USA
e-mail: gwinder@med.umich.edu

E. G. Clifton
Department of Psychiatry, University of Michigan, Ann Arbor, MI, USA
e-mail: erindef@med.umich.edu

P. Riggs, T. Thant (eds.), *Cannabis in Psychiatric Practice*, Psychiatry Update 3,
https://doi.org/10.1007/978-3-031-04874-6_17

substance use and mental health (MH). Dave presents 2 years later for transplant reevaluation after being turned down for transplant at another center for similar concerns. At the other center's recommendation, he completed an encounter of substance use disorder (SUD) treatment in his local area. He has also since begun hemodialysis secondary to his worsening kidney function.

During a subsequent interview, Dave reports his completed SUD therapy was "worthless" and reports he does not have a SUD. He is still using marijuana daily, transitioned to electronic cigarettes from tobacco, and stopped alprazolam the month prior. Toxicology and the prescription drug monitoring program both support this.

Dave accepts mirtazapine as a medication to treat anxiety and mood and possibly assist in marijuana cessation via treating any withdrawal symptoms [1]. Monthly psychotherapy sessions alongside psychiatric medication management bring about improved insight into his SUD and MH. Marijuana reduction was tracked with quantitative tetrahydrocannabinol (THC) assays and eventual cessation verified with urine drug screen timed to coincide with Dave's infrequent urination. He was transplanted 10 months later and has not since followed up with psychiatry posttransplant despite recommendations to do so. He has returned to tobacco use.

Introduction

Brief Overview of Organ Transplantation

The evaluation of prospective transplant candidates ranges from time periods of hours to years. It begins with a diagnosis of end-stage organ disease and is followed by a multidisciplinary assessment for indications and contraindications for transplant. This comprehensive effort by transplant clinicians has administrative, medical, surgical, and psychosocial components. The psychosocial assessment of recipients focuses on a patient's understanding of their condition, consent and readiness for transplant, general MH, substance use, and social support. For candidates deemed appropriate by a selection committee, the next step is a place on a national wait list, a destination which can also last hours to years depending on numerous variables about a patient's disease severity as well as donor organ availability.

During time on the wait list, patients are carefully monitored prospectively in terms of their physiology, psychology, and social circumstances remaining conducive to transplant. It is common that new or recurrent medical, surgical, and psychosocial challenges prompt new discussions by the selection committee about a patient's candidacy. As circumstances warrant, transplant listings can be placed on temporary holds or patients can be de-listed altogether, thus removing the possibility of transplant at the center that listed them. Transplant candidates regularly seek second opinions at other centers and in some circumstances can be listed at multiple transplant centers.

Transplant teams are multidisciplinary entities comprised of specialists from medicine, surgery, nursing, psychiatry, psychology, social work, and other administrative disciplines. The relationships they establish with patients are lifelong given the transplanted organs require specialized care for the duration of the patient's life, such as ongoing management of immunosuppressant medication to prevent rejection. Different organ teams have unique professional cultures and policies about lower risk MH profiles and substance use. This means that psychosocial specialists (psychology, social work, psychiatry, addiction medicine), who range from embedded teammates to unaffiliated colleagues, may care for transplant patients who are subject to differing policies about marijuana use. For example, a transplant psychologist's patient census could include two patients using marijuana on a weekly basis in similar amounts but the patient with idiopathic pulmonary fibrosis could be asked by the lung transplant team to abstain from marijuana completely while the patient with IgA nephropathy could be allowed to continue marijuana use during a kidney transplant course.

Unique Features of Transplant Patients

The context of solid organ transplantation affects how and why patients use marijuana, whether they will disclose it to their transplant clinicians, and how clinicians evaluate and understand patients' marijuana use. First, patients with end-stage disease are subject to risks of severe illness morbidity and death. This activates a person's survival instinct which can influence the ways in which they interact with transplant clinicians. Patients who desire transplant will sense that they need to appear well enough to qualify, similar to making a good first impression during a date or job interview, and they may hesitate to disclose anything that they perceive could worsen their chances, including marijuana use. These powerful psychological conditions risk that patients' true feelings, intentions, and behaviors may be unavailable or actively concealed from transplant clinicians by patients and families.

Second, transplant patients, both candidates and recipients, are often not seeking MH or SUD treatment. Many are referred to see transplant psychosocial clinicians secondary to program requirements or because of team members' concerns. Many patients do not desire a psychosocial evaluation. Psychosocial clinicians commonly hear patients say that they are unsure why they are being evaluated and that they do not need any psychiatric help. Some resent having their MH or substance use discussed at all. Additionally, many patients do not feel well physically given the gravity of their medical disease and completing an extended psychosocial interview, or series of encounters, is a challenge. Each of these overlapping possibilities affects initial and long-term patient–clinician rapport and alliance.

Third, the transplant process itself is extremely stressful for patients and families. Many end-stage medical illnesses declare themselves suddenly resulting in extreme disruption to lifestyle and MH. Patients may require multiple transplants due to unforeseen adverse events, complications, or the eventual decline of their grafts. After the initial shock of illness or its return, the ensuing phases of transplant care are each characterized by unpleasant uncertainty in terms of further health deterioration, qualifying for transplant listing or re-listing, wait list and surgery survival, and postoperative adjustments. If marijuana had been a part of a patient's regular stress management, it is likely and understandable that the patient will turn to it again during such times. Stress inherent to transplant also means that psychosocial clinicians conducting pre-transplant evaluations are not simply tasked just with assessing a patient's current MH and state of mind but also gauging how a patient might manage the inevitable adversity ahead.

Fourth, transplant evaluations not only entail the assessment of individual patients but also the stewardship of precious donor organs, which remain in short supply compared to the number of patients who need them. The stewardship of donor organs has several important components and effects. It requires that, when clinicians make their decisions, they keep in mind the hundreds or thousands of other listed patients awaiting organs who are unknown, unseen, and dispersed among many regional transplant centers. In the case of living donors, clinicians must also consider the well-being of an otherwise healthy person who heroically desires to donate. Patients become aware of their team's stewardship and may view their psychosocial clinicians as transplant gatekeepers rather than partners and advocates; this can unfavorably impact candor and alliance.

Fifth, implanting donor organs into a recipient is an extraordinary endeavor involving enormous time and resources and as such it brings about an array of powerful emotions and bonds shared among patients, families, and clinicians. This means, however, that when challenges arise, particularly if they involve stigmatized issues or factors perceived as a patient's fault (MH and SUD matters often fall into these categories), those special bonds can become sources of blame, guilt, and detachment which can disrupt essential relationships.

Finally, transplant patients are a unique population in several physical and psychological attributes which impact their interactions with MH clinicians and facilities. Pre-transplant patients commonly have high disease burden and substantial medical complexity involving multiple organ systems, specialists, and medications. Patients who are this sick may not be able to follow up regularly due to changes in mental status (i.e., hepatic encephalopathy in liver disease), frequent medical appointments or dialysis, and unexpected hospital admissions. As many MH agencies are already saturated with severely ill patients in need, any no-shows could jeopardize a patient's access to ongoing psychiatric care.

Overview and Significance of Marijuana in Organ Transplantation

Logistical, Legal, and Ethical Matters

There is significant heterogeneity across organ communities, transplant centers, teams, and clinicians with regard to marijuana policy [2–4]. There are no consensus guidelines from professional societies or governing bodies about thresholds of acceptable use or how marijuana assessments should be conducted. These factors ensure that marijuana use is among the most controversial and debated topics that transplant teams encounter [2]. The controversy of marijuana and organ transplantation has been the subject of media attention as well as legislation proscribing discrimination against patients on the basis of their marijuana use. It behooves clinicians to regard marijuana as another relevant health behavior that is no more or less important in transplant than tobacco, exercise, alcohol, sexual behavior, diet, medication adherence, herbal supplements, etc.

Clinicians sometimes use marijuana's legal status as the basis for arguments for or against its use in the transplant population [3]. This reasoning alone is insufficient given the tremendous and tragic disease burden wrought by alcohol and tobacco, two legal and widely available substances which often lead to end-stage diseases themselves requiring organ transplantation. There are also myriad harms arising from the so-called "war on drugs" in the United States, an effort which employs the legal system to influence how the population uses recreational substances. Since a SUD evaluation inevitably seeks to understand substance use in spite of severe consequences, including legal problems, marijuana's ever-evolving legal status in the United States can create confusion for transplant centers serving broad geographic regions containing jurisdictions with divergent marijuana policies.

In organ transplant, substance use and other lifestyle factors invoke key ethical principles also worth considering with regard to marijuana. The first is medical utility which is minimizing patient harm (nonmaleficence) while maximizing patient benefit, organ survival, and improved quality of life (beneficence) [5]. Applied to marijuana use, clinicians need to determine if there are direct or indirect effects, medically or psychosocially, of a patient's use that may favorably or adversely impact their transplant course. Another key ethical principle is that of justice which is that equitable and reasonable transplant practices and policies should exist for all patients [5]. Regarding marijuana use, clinicians should determine if certain individual patients or populations are being scrutinized differently or policies are being applied unfairly.

Marijuana Stigma and Idealization

Emotion and opinion within the professional and lay communities regarding marijuana are often strong. Some voices indicate medicinal value of marijuana and the stigma attached to its use while others point to substantial risks of permissive use and legalization. Society continues to work through policy and healthcare implications of the evolving marijuana landscape in the United States. This process and its uncertainty are mirrored and amplified within the transplant environment. Less is known about marijuana's favorable or unfavorable effects, if any, on patients' transplant outcomes and treatment courses due to a relative paucity of literature on the topic. Ideally, transplant clinicians apply objective guidelines and algorithms derived from medical and ethical literature to guide their clinical decision-making with regard to marijuana. The lack of such research and consensus means that it is often team culture and precedent that leads to decisions about patients' marijuana use. This leaves substantial and regrettable open space for speculation, personal experience, and strong opinion.

Transplant selection committees will inevitably have their own robust collective and individual opinions about marijuana varying widely with regard to idealism, skepticism, or pessimism. Transplant decisions are challenging at baseline given they involve end-stage disease, precious resource allocation, and the coordination of multiple medical specialties. Needed nuanced debate and careful clinical judgment with regard to marijuana use can easily be obscured by strong unchecked emotion and opinion among transplant professionals. A highly cohesive and interprofessional team culture along with tightly coordinated psychosocial evaluation procedures can facilitate fair, careful, and patient-centered decision-making in this challenging and high stakes context.

Brief Review of Existing Transplant-Specific Marijuana Literature

There are numerous biological, medical, political, and social aspects of marijuana use relevant to transplant teams [6] which are beyond the scope of this chapter. Salient attitudinal and outcome data across solid organ teams appear below.

Liver

The proportion of LT patients using marijuana is increasing [7]. In a study of pre-transplant liver transplant (LT) patients, marijuana did not associate with the probability of receiving a transplant, waitlist mortality, or delisting but was associated with alcohol-related liver disease, hepatitis C, and other substance use [8]. In another study, however, marijuana lengthened evaluations and lowered listing rates [7]. In post-LT patients, marijuana does affect survival but tends to be used by younger male patients with hepatitis C and lower Model for End-Stage Liver Disease (MELD) scores who use controlled substances [7, 9–11]. Marijuana is becoming more accepted on LT teams but only a small minority of programs transplant active marijuana users [12].

Heart and Lung

Heart and lung transplant teams perceive marijuana's legality in the patient's jurisdiction as relevant to their transplant candidacy and are more likely to support medical marijuana patients than recreational users [3, 13]. Lung donor cannabis use has both been shown to be unrelated to post-lung transplant outcomes [14] as well as implicated in poorer survival [15]. In a population of cardiac donors with a history of high-risk social behaviors, marijuana use did not associate with recipient survival [16]. THC vaping has been identified by the FDA as a particular risk of lung injury [17] which has itself led to a double lung transplant [18].

Kidney

In post-kidney transplant patients, marijuana use has been shown to have an unfavorable impact on graft failure rates in one study [19] while others show no difference in survival or graft failure rates or worse organ function [20, 21].

Marijuana may associate, however, with other psychosocial problems such as drinking, other drug use, nonadherence, and certain psychiatric disorders [21].

Potential General Benefits of Marijuana Use in Transplant Patients

Transplant patients experience neuropathic pain [22] which may be related to primary medical conditions (i.e., diabetes), substance use (i.e., alcohol), surgical procedures, or use of medications (i.e., calcineurin inhibitors). Cannabinoids have moderate-quality evidence supporting their use in chronic neuropathic pain [23] and might be effective in targeting these symptoms. As transplant patients have numerous other medical and surgical foci for pain, marijuana could represent a lower risk alternative to opioids [24]. Sleep problems also occur in transplant patients [25] and some lower-quality evidence exists that cannabinoids might be useful in their treatment [23]. End-stage disease states commonly impair appetite or cause nausea and vomiting and low-quality evidence exists that these can be improved with cannabinoids [23]. Depression and anxiety are common in many end-stage disease states [26–30] as well as in various transplant populations. While there is no evidence supporting the use of marijuana to treat such psychiatric conditions and there is only emerging evidence supporting the use of CBD for anxiety [31], many transplant patients report that these are primary conditions for which they are using marijuana. Similar to other transplant-related consultation requests, as teams develop questions about therapeutic aspects of patients' marijuana use, consult requests to relevant specialists (i.e., pain medicine, gastroenterology, neurology, psychiatry) are appropriate.

Potential General Risks of Marijuana Use in Transplant Patients

The lifestyle of end-stage disease patients and transplant recipient is demanding in terms of essential adherence to complex medication and treatment regimens. To the degree that marijuana affects a patient's cognition [32, 33], this could be a potential source of risk and morbidity in terms of nonadherence. Marijuana can be habit-forming and addictive [33]; the inherent hazards of dependency and SUD are often magnified in end-stage disease and transplant. In some patients, marijuana may actually be a cause or perpetuating factor in chronic nausea and vomiting [34, 35] with broad physiological implications in transplant patients. There are case reports of serious pulmonary infections in transplant patients arising from marijuana [36]. Cannabinoids are substrates, inhibitors, and inducers of drug metabolizing enzymes [37] and there are case reports of cannabinoids interfering with immunosuppressant medication levels with significant clinical consequences [38–40]. Varying and unpredictable content, purity, and strength of a patient's product [41, 42] along with different ways in which the drug is administered (smoking, vaping, eating, etc.) could have unpredictable effects. On a case-by-case basis and in accordance with transplant center policies, the balance of marijuana's benefits and risks should be carefully scrutinized.

Evaluating and Treating Marijuana Use in Transplant Patients

General Approach

MH and SUD evaluations within transplant have some unique attributes that are directly relevant to marijuana-related assessments. To be successful, transplant psychosocial clinicians require adept skills at rapidly establishing rapport and trust, destigmatizing MH and SUD matters, ensuring patient awareness of the broader transplant implications of the evaluation, full disclosure of evaluation confidentiality and its limits, maintaining equipoise of the risks and benefits of marijuana use, tailoring psychotherapy goals to the transplant process, adjusting pharmacological treatments to organ failure and other pharmacotherapies, and setting expectations for treatment and follow-up.

Many transplant patients are already overwhelmed by what is happening to their bodies, families, and lifestyle as a result of their illness. Anticipating and acknowledging these struggles early can build needed trust and alliance quickly during an evaluation. Clinicians need to understand the transplant process as well as patient emotions related to going through it. As patients sense that their clinician is not only aware of their situation and authentically compassionate around the distress they feel, the encounter related to marijuana use is more likely to be successful.

Many patients using marijuana are rightly sensitive to stigma and bias. Many are already habituated to under-reporting their use or concealing it altogether. Transplant clinicians should be able to elicit, acknowledge, and comprehend the reasons why patients value their marijuana use and any drawbacks or side effects patients have noticed. Similar to other substance use evaluations, there are several strategies which are of particular importance in transplant given the need to reduce sensitivity and guardedness and build rapid and enduring patient alliances: using accurate and appropriate marijuana-related vocabulary (both technical and casual), neutrally acknowledging pros and cons of marijuana use, normalizing the ubiquity of marijuana use in general and transplant populations, modeling destigmatized attitudes toward marijuana, using temperate language and a conversational tone of voice, seeking opportunities for brief and appropriate levity and humor, avoiding "gotcha" or authoritarian styles, and starting with lower intensity topics and leaving heavier discussions for the end of the encounter. The spirit and partnership of motivational interviewing [43] is an applicable and useful paradigm to marijuana discussions in transplant.

Demarcating boundaries of confidentiality is essential during the transplant evaluation's introduction. Patients should understand that what they say will remain with the clinician and medical record documentation except where written permission is obtained or emergency procedures require additional disclosure. Clinicians should understand that the amount and tone of information they place in the medical record can be read by patients, clinician colleagues, and other transplant centers with all that this implies for future treatment encounters and the patient's transplant course. Clinicians should clearly inform patients that they alone do not decide whether the patient is listed or receives an organ; transplant-related decisions are never made by a single clinician but rather by a selection committee. We find that stating MH- and SUD-related matters are "no more and no less than one slice in the transplant pie" is a useful metaphor to convey this idea.

Clinical judgment in marijuana-related matters in transplant should be guided by the literature whenever possible. Clinicians should consult marijuana-related literature inside and outside transplant, note its gaps, bias, and uncertainties, and refer to it during interactions with patients and transplant colleagues. Cautious use of psychotropic medications in patients with organ failure should be informed by manufacturer recommendations for dosing adjustments along with medical consultation. Transplant teams should be made aware of psychiatric medication changes. Medication interactions are possible with the extensive drug regimens many transplant patients require; querying databases and consulting pharmacist colleagues are important practices. Toxicology, discussed more below, is an essential tool in marijuana-related clinical work whose use and interpretation should be thoroughly discussed with patients early in the transplant process.

Psychotherapy is commonly prescribed in marijuana-using transplant patients either to address a marijuana use disorder or to treat comorbidities. As many transplant patients are not seeking MH or SUD treatment, extra work early in the treatment process to orient patients and their therapists to transplant's nuances, idiosyncrasies, and timetables mentioned above may increase chances that therapy is successful. Transplant teams often desire that marijuana patients, regardless of active MH or SUD symptoms, remain in therapy before and after transplant to minimize disorder recurrence and maximize chances that transplant-related stress is managed in a healthy manner; this should be clearly conveyed to patients and therapists.

Psychiatric and SUD Comorbidities

Given that marijuana use may correlate with psychopathology, SUD, and other unfavorable psychosocial outcomes [44–47], transplant teams should be thorough and cautious with their marijuana-related evaluations whether or not they suspect that marijuana is directly causing problems. Resulting risk profiles from careful transplant psychosocial evaluations should then guide marijuana-related recommendations. As stated above, marijuana should be understood as a health behavior on par with other behavioral variables important in transplant like diet, physical fitness, drinking, smoking, medical adherence, social support, etc. If transplant patients carry added risks in these domains, transplant teams may make additional and tailored requirements or treatment recommendations not applied to patients without said risks.

A team which permits marijuana use in its patients may opt to require full marijuana cessation in a patient with substantial psychosocial risk factors while allowing ongoing low level use in a patient without these risks. For transplant teams where marijuana use is not permitted in any patients, full cessation may be required in all patients regardless of frequency and amount of use and MH and SUD risk profiles.

After issuing recommendations, teams should check in prospectively via a treatment plan that may include clinical examinations, toxicology, psychometrics, interprofessional care coordination, and appropriate collateral information from support persons.

Psychometric Instruments

Questionnaires incrementally increase disclosure of substance use in transplant patients [48]. We find it helpful to screen all patients referred for transplant psychiatry evaluations with instruments querying mood, anxiety, sleep, drinking, and drug use. We then prospectively track relevant MH and SUD symptoms using the appropriate instruments. Electronic questionnaires are pushed to patients prior to in-person or virtual visits via the patient portal of our institution's electronic medical record. Paper questionnaires are handed to patients who are not using the portal in the waiting room prior to in-person visits. We use both electronic and paper forms to ensure we obtain data from as many patients as possible, regardless of patients' comfort with technology. We also use a clinician rating scale, the Stanford Integrated Psychosocial Assessment for Transplant (SIPAT), as an adjunctive tool to assess patients' general psychosocial suitability for transplant; marijuana and other substance use is a core part of this scale [49].

Toxicology

We are in favor of toxicological screening all patients for alcohol, drugs including marijuana, and tobacco at least once as part of a general transplant evaluation. The reasons for this include the ubiquity of substance use as well as the ethical principle of justice for all prospective candidates. Unremarkable toxicology is a pertinent negative finding similar to other unremarkable laboratory, physical examination, and imaging findings. Also, transplant may foster patient concealment, as discussed above, meaning that the clinical follow-up to positive results can yield essential substance-related conversations and insights that would have only taken place via objective toxicological data about a patient's exposure to substances. As stated above, the clinical interview following unexpected positive results must be compassionate and neutral to maintain rapport and partnership.

The American Society of Addiction Medicine (ASAM) has issued pertinent guidelines related to appropriate use of toxicology in medicine that are useful in transplant [50]. Some pertinent practices include toxicology used as a useful tool for: supporting SUD recovery rather than exacting punishment; exploring denial, motivation, and actual substance use; verifying patient clinical reports of use; and catalyzing therapeutic discussions when toxicology results contradict patient self-reports. ASAM also cautions that positive toxicology results are not sufficient for a SUD diagnosis and negative results cannot ensure that a patient has not used.

Many labs will include THC on a panel of urine immunoassays which screen for different recreational substances. Given the stakes of positive immunoassay results in transplant (i.e., evaluation closed, listings held, delisting), confirmation testing can be essential for positive results. At our institution, we have toured the toxicology lab and gotten to know some of the technicians to ensure that we can collaborate well when a positive lab test must be carefully understood and confirmed.

In patients with organ failure, metabolism and clearance of THC may be prolonged meaning patients will continue to test positive long after they have stopped using. Obtaining separate quantitative urine THC levels can be helpful in verifying ongoing abstinence as values trend downward. Most importantly, all consequential toxicology results should be discussed with patients directly relying on the partnership and compassion already established as part of a strong clinician–patient alliance.

Transplant Policy Awareness and MH/SUD Treatment Adherence

Patients should be aware of a team and/or center's marijuana policies. They should clearly understand if they will be tested for marijuana use (and other substances if indicated) as part of their transplant course and how those results will be interpreted and used by the team. Some transplant centers have patients sign substance use agreements as a documented, shared understanding as to how substance use will be evaluated and toxicology results interpreted as the transplant course continues.

When MH and SUD treatment is prescribed in transplant patients using marijuana, gauging patient adherence and treatment response is important. Transplant populations are often numerous and widely dispersed geographically meaning regular and frequent follow-up with transplant MH and SUD clinicians may not be feasible. This means that partnering with local community MH and SUD clinicians is essential. There are several helpful practices which may facilitate this partnership. Sending an introduction packet with referred patients can help introduce transplant clinicians and provide some general orientation regarding the unique facets of transplant mental health as many community partners will not have treated transplant patients before. Interval written and phone correspondence is helpful to check in on patient progress as well as guiding treatment goals to align with transplant needs. Soliciting written summary letters as treatment episodes conclude are important for documentation and for relaying information to the selection committee. Transplant center outreach activities for continuing medical education are another way to build these important treatment partnerships.

When the selection committee requires MH and SUD treatment before and/or after transplant, this should be clearly communicated with patients and their clinicians. Many transplant patients have never received such treatment before making a brief, practical orientation to the theory and practice of MH/SUD treatment helpful. Assisting patients in developing some initial treatment goals they can suggest with their new MH/SUD clinicians can also jumpstart their treatment. Transplant patients may be highly motivated to meet selection committee requirements but this will not guarantee that they progress adequately in their MH/SUD treatment. Thresholds of adequate treatment response must be assessed in case-by-case fashion while ensuring as equitable and consistent standards as possible.

Summary

There are few clear answers regarding marijuana use in transplant and significant heterogeneity in policy and attitude across transplant organ communities, teams, and clinicians. Amid such complexity, controversy, and consequence, transplant teams must maintain destigmatized attitudes, apply equitable judgment to their marijuana-using patients, trust and collaborate with their psychosocial clinician colleagues, and stay abreast of the evolving marijuana issue and literature.

Highlights Box 17.1 Key Points for Patient Psychoeducation

- Transplant teams' main goals include achieving definitive treatment of end-stage disease and improving patient quality of life; if marijuana use threatens these goals, it will likely be something a patient will be asked to address, such as a requirement to fully abstain.
- The risks and benefits of marijuana use are evaluated uniquely and thoroughly in organ transplantation due to the shortage and preciousness of donor organs.
- Despite lack of clear guidelines in the literature, transplant clinicians endeavor to communicate concerns and recommendations regarding patients' marijuana use, including encouraging patient honesty and transparency around their use.
- Transplant teams commonly use toxicological lab tests to screen and monitor marijuana use similar to how they use other tests to monitor other organs and diseases.

Highlights Box 17.2 Key Points in Treatment and Management

- No consensus exists regarding marijuana use and its evaluation in organ transplantation which increases the importance of ethical, equitable, and destigmatized clinical judgment.
- There are few data indicating marijuana associates with harm in transplant patients while data linking marijuana to other concerning and consequential psychosocial risks and variables are more prevalent.
- There are accumulating case reports of cannabinoids unfavorably interfering with immunosuppressant medications.
- Marijuana has varying risk profiles according to transplant population and dose and frequency of use.

- Transplant patients with significant mental health and substance use disorder histories could reasonably be encouraged to abstain completely from marijuana.
- Organ transplantation entails broad multidisciplinary collaboration necessitating strong teamwork and clear communication around potentially stigmatized matters like marijuana use.

References

1. Benyamina A, Lecacheux M, Blecha L, Reynaud M, Lukasiewcz M. Pharmacotherapy and psychotherapy in cannabis withdrawal and dependence. Expert Rev Neurother. 2008;8(3): 479–91.
2. Secunda K, Gordon EJ, Sohn MW, Shinkunas LA, Kaldjian LC, Voigt MD, et al. National survey of provider opinions on controversial characteristics of liver transplant candidates. Liver Transpl. 2013;19(4):395–403.
3. Neyer J, Uberoi A, Hamilton M, Kobashigawa JA. Marijuana and listing for heart transplant: a survey of transplant providers. Circ Heart Fail. 2016;9(7):e002851.
4. Pondrom S. Transplantation and marijuana use. Am J Transplant. 2016;16(1):1–2.
5. Veatch RM, Ross LF. Transplantation ethics. Washington, DC: Georgetown University Press; 2015.
6. Rai HS, Winder GS. Marijuana use and organ transplantation: a review and implications for clinical practice. Curr Psychiatry Rep. 2017;19(11):91.
7. Likhitsup A, Saeed N, Winder GS, Hassan A, Sonnenday CJ, Fontana RJ. Marijuana use among adult liver transplant candidates and recipients. Clin Transpl. 2021;35:e14312.
8. Kotwani P, Saxena V, Dodge JL, Roberts J, Yao F, Hameed BJ. History of marijuana use does not affect outcomes on the liver transplant waitlist. Transplantation. 2018;102(5):794.
9. Ranney DN, Acker WB, Al-Holou SN, Ehrlichman L, Lee DS, Lewin SA, et al. Marijuana use in potential liver transplant candidates. Am J Trasplant. 2009;9(2):280–5.
10. Serrano Rodriguez P, Strassle PD, Barritt AS IV, Watkins R, Gerber DA, Hayashi PH, et al. Marijuana consumption in liver transplant recipients. Liver Transpl. 2019;25(5):734–40.
11. Guorgui J, Ito T, Markovic D, Aziz A, Younan S, Severance A, et al. The impact of marijuana use on liver transplant recipients: a 900 patient single center experience. Clin Transplant. 2021;35:e14215.
12. Zhu J, Chen P-Y, Frankel M, Selby RR, Fong T-L. Contemporary policies regarding alcohol and marijuana use among liver transplant programs in the United States. Transplantation. 2018;102(3):433–9.
13. Phillips KA, Thrush PT, Lal AK, Kindel SJ, Castleberry C, Sparks J, et al. Marijuana in pediatric and adult congenital heart disease heart transplant listing: a survey of provider practices and attitudes. Pediatr Transplant. 2020;24(2):e13640.
14. Mohite PN, Zeriouh M, Sáez DG, Popov AF, Sabashnikov A, Zych B, et al. Influence of history of cannabis smoking in selected donors on the outcomes of lung transplantation. Eur J Cardiothorac Surg. 2017;51(1):142–7.
15. Okahara S, Levvey B, McDonald M, D'Costa R, Opdam H, Pilcher DV, et al. Influence of the donor history of tobacco and marijuana smoking on early and intermediate lung transplant outcomes. J Heart Lung Transplant. 2020;39(9):962–9.
16. Xu DS, Hartman D, Ludrosky K, Campbell J, Starling RC, Taylor DO, et al. Impact of donor high-risk social behaviors on recipient survival in cardiac transplantation. Transplantation. 2010;89(7):873–8.

17. Vaping Illness update: FDA warns public to stop using tetrahydrocannabinol (THC)-containing vaping products and any vaping products obtained off the street. https://www.fda.gov/consumers/consumer-updates/vaping-illness-update-fda-warns-public-stop-using-tetrahydrocannabinol-thc-containing-vaping.
18. Nemeh H, Coba V, Chulkov M, Gupta A, Yeldo N, Chamogeorgakis T, et al. Lung transplantation for the treatment of vaping induced, irreversible, end stage lung injury. Ann Thorac Surg. 2021;111:e353.
19. Vaitla PK, Thongprayoon C, Hansrivijit P, Kanduri SR, Kovvuru K, Rivera FHC, et al. Epidemiology of cannabis use and associated outcomes among kidney transplant recipients: a meta-analysis. J Evid Based Med. 2021;14:90.
20. Greenan G, Ahmad SB, Anders MG, Leeser A, Bromberg JS, Niederhaus SV. Recreational marijuana use is not associated with worse outcomes after renal transplantation. Clin Transpl. 2016;30(10):1340–6.
21. Alhamad T, Koraishy FM, Lam NN, Katari S, Naik AS, Schnitzler MA, et al. Cannabis dependence or abuse in kidney transplantation: implications for posttransplant outcomes. Transplantation. 2019;103(11):2373–82.
22. Öcal R, Tanoğlu C, Kibaroğlu S, Derle E, Can U, Kirnap M, et al. Prevalence and treatment of neuropathic pain in kidney and liver transplant recipients Exp Clin Transplant. 2017. https://doi.org/10.6002/ect.2016.0151
23. Whiting PF, Wolff RF, Deshpande S, Di Nisio M, Duffy S, Hernandez AV, et al. Cannabinoids for medical use: a systematic review and meta-analysis. JAMA. 2015;313(24):2456–73.
24. Bachhuber MA, Saloner B, Cunningham CO, Barry CL. Medical cannabis laws and opioid analgesic overdose mortality in the United States, 1999-2010. JAMA Intern Med. 2014;174(10):1668–73.
25. Cheng E, Evangelidis N, Guha C, Hanson CS, Unruh M, Wilkie M, et al. Patient experiences of sleep in dialysis: systematic review of qualitative studies. Sleep Med. 2021;80:66–76.
26. Easton K, Coventry P, Lovell K, Carter L-A, Deaton C. Prevalence and measurement of anxiety in samples of patients with heart failure: meta-analysis. J Cardiovasc Nurs. 2016;31(4):367.
27. Peng T, Hu Z, Guo L, Xia Q, Li D, Yang X. Relationship between psychiatric disorders and quality of life in nondialysis patients with chronic kidney disease. Am J Med Sci. 2013;345(3):218–21.
28. Sumanathissa M, De Silva VA, Hanwella R. Prevalence of major depressive episode among patients with pre-dialysis chronic kidney disease. Int J Psychiatry Med. 2011;41(1):47–56.
29. Cron D, Friedman J, Winder G, Thelen A, Derck J, Fakhoury J, et al. Depression and frailty in patients with end-stage liver disease referred for transplant evaluation. 2016;16(6):1805–11.
30. Matte DL, Pizzichini MM, Hoepers AT, Diaz AP, Karloh M, Dias M, et al. Prevalence of depression in COPD: a systematic review and meta-analysis of controlled studies. Respir Med. 2016;117:154–61.
31. Blessing EM, Steenkamp MM, Manzanares J, Marmar CR. Cannabidiol as a potential treatment for anxiety disorders. Neurotherapeutics. 2015;12(4):825–36.
32. Auer R, Vittinghoff E, Yaffe K, Kunzi A, Kertesz SG, Levine DA, et al. Association between lifetime marijuana use and cognitive function in middle age: the coronary artery risk development in young adults (CARDIA) study. JAMA Intern Med. 2016;176(3):352–61.
33. Volkow ND, Compton WM, Weiss SR. Adverse health effects of marijuana use. N Engl J Med. 2014;371(9):879.
34. Kim HS, Anderson JD, Saghafi O, Heard KJ, Monte AA. Cyclic vomiting presentations following marijuana liberalization in Colorado. Acad Emerg Med. 2015;22(6):694–9.
35. Allen J, De Moore G, Heddle R, Twartz J. Cannabinoid hyperemesis: cyclical hyperemesis in association with chronic cannabis abuse. Gut. 2004;53(11):1566–70.
36. Marks WH, Florence L, Lieberman J, Chapman P, Howard D, Roberts P, et al. Successfully treated invasive pulmonary aspergillosis associated with smoking marijuana in a renal transplant recipient. Trasplantation. 1996;61(12):1771–4.
37. Stout SM, Cimino NM. Exogenous cannabinoids as substrates, inhibitors, and inducers of human drug metabolizing enzymes: a systematic review. Drug Metab Rev. 2014;46(1):86–95.

38. Moadel D, Chism K. Medical marijuana-induced tacrolimus toxicity. Psychomatics. 2019;60:603–5.
39. Hauser N, Sahai T, Richards R, Roberts T. High on cannabis and calcineurin inhibitors: a word of warning in an era of legalized marijuana. Case Rep Transplant. 2016;2016:4028492.
40. Leino AD, Emoto C, Fukuda T, Privitera M, Vinks AA, Alloway RR. Evidence of a clinically significant drug-drug interaction between cannabidiol and tacrolimus. Am J Trasplant. 2019;19(10):2944–8.
41. McLaren J, Swift W, Dillon P, Allsop S. Cannabis potency and contamination: a review of the literature. Addiction. 2008;103(7):1100–9.
42. ElSohly MA, Mehmedic Z, Foster S, Gon C, Chandra S, Church JC. Changes in cannabis potency over the last 2 decades (1995–2014): analysis of current data in the United States. Biol Psychiatry. 2016;79(7):613–9.
43. Miller WR, Rollnick S, Ebook L. Motivational interviewing: helping people change. New York: Guilford Press; 2013. 1 online resource (xii, 482p).
44. McHugh M, McGorry P, Yung A, Lin A, Wood S, Hartmann J, et al. Cannabis-induced attenuated psychotic symptoms: implications for prognosis in young people at ultra-high risk for psychosis. Psychol Med. 2017;47(4):616–26.
45. Ranganathan M, Skosnik PD, D'Souza DC. Marijuana and madness: associations between cannabinoids and psychosis. Biol Psychiatry. 2016;79(7):511–3.
46. Volkow ND, Swanson JM, Evins AE, DeLisi LE, Meier MH, Gonzalez R, et al. Effects of cannabis use on human behavior, including cognition, motivation, and psychosis: a review. JAMA Psychiatry. 2016;73(3):292–7.
47. Compton WM, Han B, Jones CM, Blanco C, Hughes A. Marijuana use and use disorders in adults in the USA, 2002–14: analysis of annual cross-sectional surveys. Lancet Psychiatry. 2016;3(10):954–64.
48. Donnadieu-Rigole H, Olive L, Nalpas B, Winter A, Ursic-Bedoya J, Faure S, et al. Follow-up of alcohol consumption after liver transplantation: interest of an addiction team? Alcohol Clin Exp Res. 2017;41(1):165–70.
49. Maldonado JR, Dubois HC, David EE, Sher Y, Lolak S, Dyal J, et al. The Stanford Integrated Psychosocial Assessment for Transplantation (SIPAT): a new tool for the psychosocial evaluation of pre-transplant candidates. Psychosomatics. 2012;53(2):123–32.
50. Jarvis M, Williams J, Hurford M, Lindsay D, Lincoln P, Giles L, et al. Appropriate use of drug testing in clinical addiction medicine. J Addict Med. 2017;11(3):163–73.

Index

P. Riggs, T. Thant (eds.), *Cannabis in Psychiatric Practice*, Psychiatry Update 3,
https://doi.org/10.1007/978-3-031-04874-6

GPSR Compliance

The European Union's (EU) General Product Safety Regulation (GPSR) is a set of rules that requires consumer products to be safe and our obligations to ensure this.

If you have any concerns about our products, you can contact us on ProductSafety@springernature.com

In case Publisher is established outside the EU, the EU authorized representative is:

Springer Nature Customer Service Center GmbH
Europaplatz 3
69115 Heidelberg, Germany

Batch number: 10726135

Printed by Printforce, the Netherlands